Health Promotion
for
Pharmacists

Alison Blenkinsopp

Director, Centre for Pharmacy
Postgraduate Education, Manchester

Rhona Panton

Regional Pharmaceutical Officer
West Midlands Regional Health Authority

Oxford   New York   Tokyo
OXFORD UNIVERSITY PRESS
1991

Oxford University Press, Walton Street, Oxford OX2 6DP

Oxford New York Toronto
Delhi Bombay Calcutta Madras Karachi
Petaling Jaya Singapore Hong Kong Tokyo
Nairobi Dar es Salaam Cape Town
Melbourne Auckland
and associated companies in
Berlin Ibadan

Oxford is a trade mark of Oxford University Press

Published in the United States
by Oxford University Press, New York

British Library Cataloguing in Publication Data
A catalogue record for this book is available from the British Library

Library of Congress Cataloging in Publication Data
Blenkinsopp, Alison.
Health promotion for pharmacists/Alison Blenkinsopp, Rhona
Panton.
p. cm.—(Oxford medical publications)
Includes bibliographical references and index.
1. Health counseling. 2. Pharmacist and patient. I. Panton,
Rhona. II. Title. III. Series.
[DNLM: 1. Health Promotion. 2. Patient Education.
3. Pharmaceutical Services. 4. Primary Prevention. 5. Risk
Factors. WA 108 B647h]
RS92.B54 1991 610'.71–dc20 91-3014

ISBN 0-19-263009-1 (Pbk)

Photoset by Rowland Phototypesetting Ltd
Bury St Edmunds, Suffolk
Printed in Great Britain by Biddles Ltd
Guildford & King's Lynn

Preface

During the last decade, the role that the pharmacist has to play in health promotion has become widely recognized. The 'Pharmacy Healthcare' scheme in the UK distributes leaflets on health promotion from pharmacies throughout the country and is now supported by core government funding in recognition of the contribution the pharmacist has to make. Community pharmacists are taking up the opportunities offered by an extended role where they play a greater and active part in preventing ill-health and maintaining good health.

Against this background, the aim of our book is to explore health promotion from the pharmacy viewpoint as an introduction to the field of health promotion for pharmacists. Beginning with a consideration of the historical background and development of the field, we then examine the particular challenges faced by pharmacists as health educators and promoters. The complexities and difficulties of persuading members of the public to adopt healthier behaviours are addressed, with suggestions for achieving change. At the end of the book there are lists for further reading and contact points for information.

The social and behavioural aspects of health promotion must, of course, be underpinned by the scientific knowledge base of health promotion. We discuss the major health issues of today, their causes and the advice that pharmacists could offer their customers. The word 'customer' does not encapsulate the relationship between the pharmacist and the people who visit the pharmacy, because customers and consumers are generally associated fundamentally with commercial transactions; nor does 'client' provide a fully acceptable answer. In the context of health promotion, where the pharmacist is often dealing with healthy people, the word 'patient' does not have the right connotations either. We have therefore used all these terms interchangeably throughout the book.

Because we want this book to provide practical ideas about information, action, and advice for pharmacists to think about, we have included case studies wherever possible, with questions based on those asked in actual practice together with our suggestions for possible courses of action. We have discussed these with practising pharmacists and included their suggestions.

This is the first book to look at health promotion from the pharmacist's viewpoint and, more particularly, with specific reference to community pharmacy practice. Each chapter has been reviewed by an expert in the field to ensure its currency and relevance. We hope the book will help you to develop your professional practice in this exciting area.

Bradford   A.B.
August 1990   R.P.

Acknowledgements

First of all we would like to thank all the experts who reviewed individual chapters and contributed additional ideas. They were:

Chapter 1—Dr David Player, Director of Public Health, South Birmingham Health Authority;

Chapter 2—Mr Michael Burden, District Pharmaceutical Officer, Leicester and Chairman, Health Education Authority Pharmacy Advisory Group and Mr Alan Nathan, Community Pharmacy Teacher-Practitioner and member, Health Education Authority Primary Care Advisory Group;

Chapter 3—Dr Norman Morrow, Director of Continuing Pharmaceutical Education for Northern Ireland;

Chapter 4—Ms Lynn Stockley, Head of Nutrition Education, Health Education Authority;

Chapter 5—Mrs Joy Wingfield, Law Department, Royal Pharmaceutical Society of Great Britain;

Chapter 6—Miss Elizabeth Skinner, Head of Education, Cancer Research Campaign;

Chapter 7—Miss Amanda Sandford, Head of Information, Action on Smoking and Health;

Chapter 8—Dr Ifhtar Akhtar, Consultant Psychiatrist, West Birmingham Health Authority;

Chapter 9—Ms Maggie Sanderson, Senior Lecturer in Dietetics Polytechnic of North London;

Chapter 10—Mrs Margaret Ade, H.V. Cert., RSCN, RGN, Health Visitor, Meanwood Health Centre, Leeds;

Chapter 11—Ms Toni Belfield, Head of Information, Family Planning Association;

Chapter 12—Mrs Kay Roberts, Deputy Chief Pharmacist, Welsh Office; Mrs Joy Wingfield, Law Department, Royal Pharmaceutical Society of Great Britain and Mrs Sue Lunec, Pharmacist Co-ordinator, West Midlands Regional Syringe Needle Exchange Scheme.

This book would never have been produced without the help of the many West Midlands community pharmacists who freely gave their time and advice to the several research projects in health promotion which form its basis. These projects were funded by the West Midlands Regional Advisory Group on Health Promotion. Special thanks are due to Dr Michael Harrison, Regional Medical Officer and Dr John Beasley, Regional Specialist in Public Health Medicine for their constant encouragement, interest in, and enthusiasm for extending the role of the community pharmacist in health promotion.

We are grateful to the following organizations for providing us with relevant statistical information and giving permission for data to be included:

The Cancer Research Campaign, for its factsheets with statistics on incidence, prevalence, morbidity and mortality from cancer;

The Coronary Prevention Group, for statistics from its database;

Staff at the library of the Royal Pharmaceutical Society of Great Britain helped us to locate many references, as did Dr Barry Strickland-Hodge.

Ron Morley typed the manuscript with endless patience and care and contributed many ideas in the process.

Sarah Coleman produced the artwork for Chapter 1.

Contents

To John and Howard, with love

1 What is health promotion?

When asked to identify those factors which have made the greatest impact on health in the last century, many pharmacists, like other health professionals, will cite the introduction of vaccination programmes and the discovery of antibiotics. In fact the reduction of mortality from the major killer diseases of the nineteenth and early twentieth century began long before the advent of either vaccination or antibiotics.

The factors which played the largest part in improving health were societal changes, particularly the introduction of legislation to improve living conditions and sanitation, and the creation of the Welfare State.

This chapter will review the history of the changing health of the population since the mid-nineteenth century and will address some of the key issues in health promotion today. The social, political, personal, and medical factors which influence our health will be discussed. This background is essential for pharmacists to understand the context of the health promotion activities and advice which they might offer.

1.1 What is health?

Health means different things to different people and many attempts have been made to define it. Health is:

A state of complete physical, mental and social well-being and not merely the absence of disease or infirmity (World Health Organization 1947)

A state of optimum capacity for effective performance of valued tasks (Parsons 1979)

The expression of the extent to which the individual and the social body maintain in readiness the resources to meet the exigencies of the future (Dubos 1962)

A relative state that represents the degree to which an individual can operate effectively within the circumstances of his heredity and his physical and cultural environment (McDermott 1977)

These definitions suggest that health should not be thought of purely on the basis of physical fitness or the lack of identifiable disease. The concept of a holistic approach to health, where the whole person and not simply the working parts of the body are considered, has gained increasing acceptance in recent years. Health professionals learn about their work almost exclusively in terms of diagnosis of diseases and their management and treatment. However, a person's attitudes, background, education, and culture will all contribute to their beliefs about health. As pharmacists we should be aware that health involves more than pathology and therapeutics, but involves psychological and sociological issues.

1.2 What is health promotion?

The term **Health education** is normally used to describe activities which are designed to extend the knowledge of individuals about the maintenance of good health and the prevention of ill-health. **Health promotion** is now commonly considered to have a wider meaning, incorporating health education and additionally addressing societal and governmental influence and necessary changes.

Primary prevention is concerned with preventing specific diseases developing in individuals. The efforts of primary health promotion are directed at healthy individuals, with the aim of preventing ill-health and positively improving the quality of life. Activities may include vaccination and immunization, the reduction of specific behaviours which cause disease (particularly smoking), and encouragement of general behaviour which is known to reduce health risks (for example, taking more exercise). Traditionally, health promotion and education have been most strongly identified with primary prevention.

Secondary prevention is concerned with stimulating people to respond to services for the early detection and treatment of diseases once they are established and to ensure that those treated recognize how best they can cooperate and assist with their treatment. Sometimes it may be possible to prevent the disease progressing to an irreversible stage and secondary prevention aims to return the individual to good health. Activities might include direct patient education and screening, for example cervical and breast cancer screening programmes. When disease states occur they do not always present with symptoms, and in these cases routine screening may be of benefit, for example the detection of congenital abnormalities in the fetus and of hypertension in adults.

Tertiary prevention ensures that patients respond effectively where the condition or disease cannot be completely cured. This aims to ensure that the individual is helped after diagnosis or treatment to limit the recurrence of the disease, minimize disability, and return to as active a life as possible. Education about rehabilitation may be equally directed towards ex-patients and their relatives.

Health promotion activities may be designed to be effective through three specific target audiences:

1. patients and groups of patients, or individuals and groups who may become patients;

2. health services and other staff concerned with the provision of services and coordinating the efforts of staff from different disciplines;

3. local and national government where changes may be required.

It is, however, important to remember that health promotion programmes can have a great impact on people's lives and that such programmes should always be evaluated to assess their benefits, disadvantages, and effectiveness. The possibility of adverse effects from any preventive measure or treatment must be set against the danger of severe illness or even death from the disease itself. Health promotion activities should present a concerned person with current information about the relative risks and benefits so that an informed decision can be made.

Having considered definitions of health and the concept of health promotion, we shall now look back to the nineteenth century and describe the changes in knowledge and action in relation to health which set the scene for today's health problems and activities.

1.3 The public health movement in Victorian England (1840–1900)

The health status of most people changed very little from prehistory to the middle of the nineteenth century. Prior to the Victorian age, poverty was part of the natural order of things. In Victorian times poverty was seen as an individual problem (the product of a deficient personal character and morality) and the poor were seen as thriftless, lazy, and undisciplined, lacking initiative and moral fibre. While the poor were to be assisted in coping with their condition of poverty, any improvement had to be achieved through their own efforts. The famous 'self-help' movement of the Victorian era was based on the premise that people were poor as a result of their own faults.

Then, as now, however, poverty was created by the economic arrangements and relationships of society which in turn determined the distribution of material resources. Power and wealth were concentrated in one sector. In a society where effective political organization was outlawed, people worked long hours in what we would now consider to be horrific conditions and for low wages. The Poor Laws were devised with the work ethic in mind: while relief would be given to the needy, the conditions would be so harsh as to deter most—for example by consigning them to workhouses or orphanages. The uptake of poor relief is, therefore, an inaccurate estimate of the real social conditions of those times. Of those who applied for poor relief in 1842, the reasons included insufficient wages (20 per cent), sickness (40 per cent), and old age (50 per cent). More than one reason may have been cited when claiming poor relief, hence the percentages totalling more than 100.

Against this background, crusading efforts were made to improve working-class living conditions, partly as a result of the endeavours of charismatic figures like Edwin Chadwick who, as secretary of the Poor Law Commission in the 1830s, continued to support segregation of the needy into workhouses but at the same time advocated free elementary schooling and better sanitary standards.

Sanitary reform was essential because the fast-developing cities still relied for waste disposal and clean water on the principles which had worked in rural England, in which there was a plentiful supply of fresh water and excrement was spread on the fields. In Victorian cities, excrement flowed down open sewers and inevitably contaminated fresh water supplies. Water-borne infectious diseases such as typhoid were endemic.

There was a widespread belief that these diseases were caused by 'miasma', or bad air, and Chadwick's belief that they were water-borne was given little credence. In 1836, as a result of his efforts, death certificates began to state the cause of death and Chadwick produced 'sanitary maps' showing that most death and disease occurred in overcrowded areas and that mortality was clearly related to social class. At this time the average life expectancy was 43 years for 'gentry' and 22 years for 'labourers'. Chadwick's *Survey of the labouring population of Great Britain* in 1842 was sufficiently comprehensive to include engineering plans showing how to build and run sewage farms and how to obtain clean water from agricultural areas. Chadwick was one of the first epidemiologists—relating diseases and their distribution to identify possible causes.

Some cities—notably Liverpool—acted immediately to improve sanitation, but most waited for the Public Health Act of 1848, which made the provisions of the Act mandatory, the stimulus being a panic engendered by an epidemic of cholera. Towns and cities were required to build drains and sewers, to pave streets, and to provide clean water. A further cholera epidemic in 1849, in which 70 000 people died, acted as an additional stimulus for the establishment of Medical Officers of Health who would in future ensure compliance with the provisions of the Act.

There was still no scientific evidence that disease was spread by unclean water, and in 1854 Chadwick was sacked for his crusading vigour, a leader in *The Times* the same year expressing the view that 'we prefer to take our chance of cholera than to be bullied into health'. But evidence became available when a London doctor, John Snow, traced cholera deaths to a water pump in Golden Square. There were 600 deaths in that district, of which 344 occurred in 4 days, among those who drew water from this single pump. Snow traced the pipelines of various water companies and showed that one set was infected and when the pipes of different companies were laid side by side, that part of the population served by the infected supply contracted the disease while those on the other side of the same street did not. In his report, Snow came close to anticipating Pasteur's theory of 'germs', but further time elapsed before the theory gained widespread support.

The Public Health Act of 1875 was based on the recommendations of John Simon, the Medical Officer of Health in London. This
Act set standards of sewerage, controlled adulterants in food,
established the quarantining of infectious diseases, and decreed the
provision of infirmaries. Such legislation was justified retrospec-
tively by the breakthrough of bacteriology in 1882, which was the
beginning of medicine as a science and of disease being seen as
requiring community as well as individual action. The growing
power of the state made legislation easier to enforce and its success,
when enacted, further increased that power. Health became a
symbol of justice and equality, replacing the concept that ill-health
was an 'Act of God' on the unworthy.

The identification of causative organisms led to vaccination programmes to control infectious disease and, in the case of smallpox
and diphtheria, these were significant in reducing mortality. For
other diseases the picture is neither so clear nor so obvious as one
would imagine. Consider the case of tuberculosis, where it was
widely believed that the advent of chemotherapy and a vaccination
programme were responsible for its eradication. Figure 1.1 shows
that the incidence of the disease was declining before either of those
measures was introduced. Some have argued that the tuberculosis
organism may have mutated or in some way become less virulent.
This is possible but unlikely, since tuberculosis had been endemic in
Britain for centuries. Since the conditions of exposure to the disease
had not changed and the slums in the early years of the nineteenth
century were conducive to its spread, the strong possibility remains
that improved nutrition was the factor which influenced the down-
ward trend.

The nutritional staus of the population gradually improved after
the agricultural revolution. Previously there had been 'lean' years
following bad harvests, and starving people are much more suscept-
ible to disease. This is illustrated by the severe typhus epidemics,
the last of which occurred in Britain in 1846–8 in the aftermath of
the Irish potato famine. An improvement in diet has been postulated as a reason for the decreasing mortality of this period.

Historical analysis had demonstrated that scarlet fever has shown
four cycles of severity followed by remission (see Fig. 1.2), and
these seem to have been largely independent of environmental
conditions but due to a change in the virulence of the infective
organism. From being a major killer in the early years of this

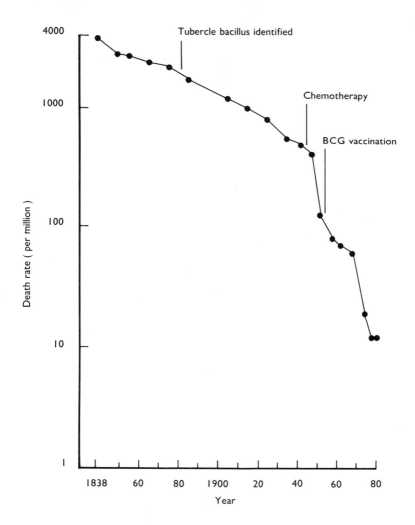

Fig. 1.1 Mean annual death rate from tuberculosis, 1838–1980. (Source: *Health, society and medicine—an introduction to community medicine*, Blackwell Scientific Publications).

century, the disease is now relatively mild, with few adverse effects. In the same way, it is thought plague and leprosy have died out in developed countries.

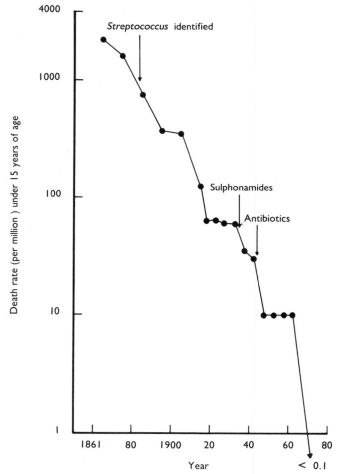

Fig. 1.2 Mean annual death rates from scarlet fever in children under 15, 1861–1980. (Source: *Health, society and medicine—an introduction to community medicine*, Blackwell Scientific Publications).

Calculations show that, in the period 1838–1900, the decrease in mortality was due to the control or eradication of diseases in the following order:

Disease state	Percentage of total decrease in mortality
Tuberculosis (respiratory)	17.5%
Cholera, dysentery, and diarrhoea	10.8%
Bronchitis, pneumonia, influenza	9.9%
Scarlet fever and diphtheria	6.2%
Typhus and typhoid	6.0%
Smallpox	1.6%

To summarize, in the nineteenth and early twentieth century there were few effective therapies, and much of the decline in mortality from disease was the result of preventive measures such as the Public Health Acts and vaccination programmes. While social factors such as an improvement in diet seem to have played a part, malnutrition was still a serious problem. At the turn of the century poverty, bad housing, and lack of provision for sickness and old age remained widespread.

1.4 Factors in better health 1900–47

While mortality from infectious diseases was declining by 1900, large differences remained in the rate of decline from different social groups, occupational classes, and comparative age groups. The infant mortality rate, for example, had not begun to fall by the end of the nineteenth century.

During the nineteenth century, little attention had been paid to such disparities, but two studies published at the turn of the century showed that most ill-health was suffered by the poor and that child health was the worst of all. In 1900, one study showed that only 2.5 per cent of the population claimed Poor Relief but other surveys carried out at that time showed the reality—that one in three people were living below the poverty line.

Booth, who carried out much research into the effects of poverty, proposed a 'poverty line' below which it was impossible to provide adequate nutrition, and for the one-third of his sample who fell below it there were four main reasons:

1. inadequate or irregular earnings;

2. large family size (22 per cent);

3. sickness (30 per cent);

4. old age (50 per cent).

More than one reason might apply, hence percentages totalling more than 100.

These findings were confirmed by an Inter-Departmental Committee on Physical Deterioration which was set up by the Government after one-half of the young men who volunteered for Boer War service were rejected due to ill-health and unsatisfactory physique. The findings were published in 1904 and revealed that over one-third of children were malnourished.

Radical changes to tackle the problems of poverty and inequality

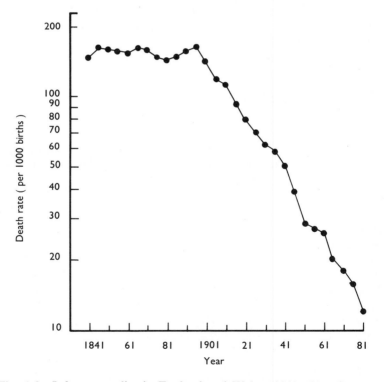

Fig. 1.3 Infant mortality in England and Wales, 1841–1981. (Source: *Health, society and medicine—an introduction to community medicine*, Blackwell Scientific Publications).

were proposed by Sidney and Beatrice Webb in a minority report on the evidence submitted to the Royal Commission on the Poor Laws, which sat from 1905 to 1909. They urged the development of welfare services to attempt to remove the poor from dependence on Poor Relief. This proposal was carried into legislation which provided meals in schools (1906), and gave a pension to old people (1908). The National Insurance Act of 1911 gave some protection against sickness to working people, and the setting up of Labour Exchanges sought to alleviate unemployment. Further legislation required notification of diseases such as tuberculosis and venereal disease, and the Maternal and Child Health Act ensured the provision of maternity care, cheap infant food, health visiting, and school health service. The fall in the infant mortality rate which occurred from the mid-eighteenth century is illustrated in Fig. 1.3.

Three factors, then, were significant in changing the health status of the nation from Victorian times to the present day:

1. public health measures, which have resulted in a clean water supply, an efficient sewage system, and a vaccination programme for the whole population;

2. fairer distribution of wealth, largely brought about by the political organization of working people;

3. a higher standard of education and knowledge of the factors which contribute to disease, which made more people aware of the ways in which they can improve their life chances.

1.5 Current inequalities in health

The Health Service Act of 1947 offered medical care to all, irrespective of economic status or geographical background. It was believed that the National Health Service would eradicate the differences in health which had previously existed. Although it seems hard to believe today, at the time of the inception of the NHS it was widely thought that the pool of existing disease would be dealt with in a year or two. Having eradicated or cured existing disease it was thought that the NHS would cost little to operate. In fact the National Health Service has consumed ever-increasing amounts of resources, and despite the original hopes the reality is that children of manual workers with large families, low incomes, and poor housing are still more likely to suffer ill-health and infant mortality than are those born of middle-class parents. Inequalities in health still remain and some experts claim that the gulf between the affluent and the poor in health terms grows ever wider.

In 1969 a National Child Development study compared children from 'ordinary' families with those from socially-disadvantaged backgrounds (children from large or single-parent families who lived in poor housing conditions on low wages).

The main findings were that children from disadvantaged backgrounds were:

1. Less likely to be protected from disease, partly because their parents did not use the immunization and screening services of the NHS.

2. More likely to have accidents in the home. This was seen as the result of overcrowding and lack of basic facilities where, for example, the boiling kettle might be the only source of hot water in the house and a paraffin heater the only source of heat.

3. Absent from school more often.

4. More likely to die in early infancy. Over the past 100 years the overall infant mortality rate has fallen from over 150 to about 15 per 1000 live births, but the relative gap between the higher and lower social classes has changed little. Approximately 30 per 1000 live births of children of unskilled backgrounds die compared with approximately 10 per 1000 live births of children born to upper-middle-class families.

For any society, research has clearly shown that the most socially disadvantaged have a health status significantly lower than the average. An awareness of this fact in situations where medical solutions are sought for what are in fact social problems helps in an assessment of how and when to offer advice on better health. When a problem is defined as an illness it becomes individual and blinds us to the more uncomfortable and harder truths of underlying social problems such as high unemployment and bad housing.

1.5.1 Inequalities in health in the 1980s and 1990s

During the 1980s two major reports were published on the subject of inequalities in health in the UK. The first of these is the *Black report*, which was published in 1980 following a working group on Inequalities in Health set up in 1977 by the Secretary of State. The conclusions of the working group were that, far from inequalities in health in the UK diminishing, they were actually increasing and that only a major and wide-ranging programme of public expenditure could set right the deep-rooted causes of those inequalities. The Government stated that the recommendations in the *Black report* regarding public spending could not be implemented and refused to endorse them.

The health divide was the second major report and was published by the then Health Education Council in 1987 just before its demise. The report was written with the aim of reviewing research and statistics on inequalities in health, drawing together and summarizing the most recent evidence. Concluding that serious social inequalities in health had persisted into the 1980s, the report stated that there was strong evidence of the major impact on health of socioeconomic circumstances. Using any measure of social standing, from the traditional social class categorization to more recent measures of deprivation, those at the bottom of the social scale had higher death rates and worse physical and mental health than those higher up. The numbers of stillbirths and of deaths in infants aged under one year continued to show a clear trend with the highest rates in social classes IV and V; deaths among adults showed a similar gradient (see Fig. 1.4).

In order to understand the evidence on social class (sometimes called occupational class) and health, the traditional categories defined by the Registrar General are as follows:

- Social class I—professional (e.g. doctor, lawyer, accountant);
- Social class II—intermediate/managerial (e.g. teacher, nurse, manager);
- Social class IIIN—skilled non-manual (e.g. typist, shop assistant);
- Social class IIIM—skilled manual (e.g. miner, bus driver, cook);
- Social class IV—semi or partly-skilled manual (e.g. farm worker, bus conductor);
- Social class V—unskilled manual (e.g. labourer, cleaner).

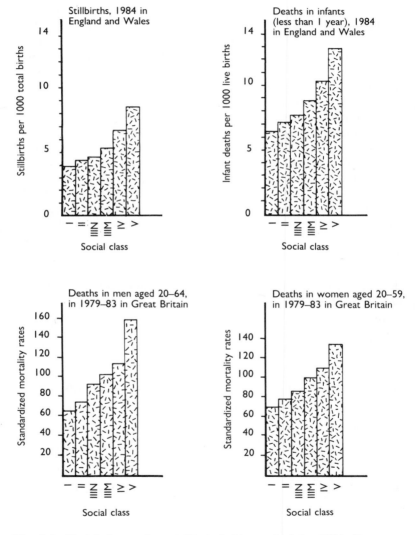

Fig. 1.4 Social class and mortality in babies and adults, 1984. (Source: OPCS 1986).

The intention of this classification was to group people together who had similar living conditions and standards. The categories were intended to reflect the level of wealth or poverty and the culture associated with each 'class'. Today, the classification is no longer seen as a precise measure but is still useful as a general guide for social position. Other measures of socioeconomic status have since been devised which take into account, for example, car and house ownership and employment status.

Both the *Black report* and *The health divide* confirmed the existence of regional differences in death rates in Great Britain. Death rates were highest in Scotland and the north and north-west of England and lowest in the south-east of England and East Anglia. Studies had clearly shown the great inequalities in health existing between neighbouring communities and the existence of pockets of poor health corresponding to areas of social and material deprivation. The adverse influence of unemployment on health was now established through research and the national gradient of unemployment—a higher level of unemployment in the north of the country was responsible for some of the ill-health.

Socioeconomic factors, while undoubtedly a major influence on health, do not explain all regional differences in morbidity and mortality. It is known that climate plays a part in health, for example ischaemic heart disease is adversely affected by cold and humidity. However, there are still large differences in morbidity and mortality from some diseases for which no explanation has yet been found—for example cancer of the stomach is 30 per cent more likely occur in parts of Wales than in England, and the incidence of spina bifida in south Wales is among the highest in the world.

Urbanization affects disease patterns and the incidence of respiratory diseases rises in cities, partly because of increased risk of infection in crowded places and partly because of the increased pollution of the atmosphere. Occupation may affect health, but the statistics can lead to inappropriate conclusions being drawn. Experts have argued that mortality statistics for coalminers are deceptively low because workers whose health has been damaged by such work will be likely to move on to other, lighter work. Allowing for these problems, occupational health statistics can teach us a great deal about the stresses and problems of various jobs—not just the newsworthy ones of asbestos workers with damaged lungs but also the physical and 'temptation' hazards of different jobs, for example publicans have a mortality rate from cirrhosis of the liver which is eight times the national average.

In adult life, morbidity and mortality from most diseases rises with social class number, so that unskilled manual workers in social class V have the highest incidence of ill-health. There are few exceptions to this trend, one being the incidence of malignant melanoma, a form of skin cancer. This serious and potentially fatal condition now occurs more frequently in higher social classes and it has been postulated that this may be due to more frequent holidays in sunny climates. Breast cancer is also found more often in those from the higher social classes.

Inequality in health between groups of differing socioeconomic status is one of the most urgent issues to be addressed, and the reduction of this inequality is the first of the WHO's (World Health Organization) European targets for Health For All. The aim is that, by the year 2000, health inequalities should be reduced by 25 per cent.

1.6 Human behaviour as a cause of disease

The endemic infectious diseases of Victorian days are now largely controlled by better living conditions, vaccination, and antibiotics. Our environment has been rendered safer by legislation such as the Factories Acts to provide safer working conditions, firm application of the drink/driving laws, and improved living standards such as the wider availability of central heating in public housing where paraffin heaters were previously the cause of many fires. These changes have resulted in fewer accidents at work, in a commendably high standard of road safety (the UK has the lowest death rate from road accidents in the EEC), and in fewer accidents in the home.

This has thrown into sharp focus the diseases for which there are, as yet, no cures. For example, AIDS and some cancers (such as lung, large bowel, and breast cancer). While lung cancer death rates are falling among men, they are still increasing among women over 55 years. Despite many years' research and vast expenditure, cures for the major cancer killers seem little nearer. Table 1.1 shows the statistics of major causes of death in the UK.

Table 1.1 Causes of death in the UK, 1987

Coronary heart disease	178 178
Cancer	160 661
Respiratory disease	66 137
Stroke	79 493
All other causes	159 882

1.6.1 The links between lifestyle and disease

Much research has focused on human behaviour as a cause of disease—that is to say, looking at individual lifestyles to see which behaviours may lead to ill-health. While individual behaviour undoubtedly contributes to the development of some diseases, it is accepted that government action is needed to bring about widespread change. The example of seat-belt legislation is often quoted in this context. Before the introduction of legislation on the wearing of seat-belts large numbers of people were killed or injured each year in road accidents. Extensive advertising campaigns and exhortations to change personal behaviour were unsuccessful and the desired behaviour change was finally achieved by legislation. In the nineteenth century water-borne diseases were not eradicated by encouraging individuals to boil water but by state legislation.

The behaviours which are harmful to health and which we will go on to discuss now and later in this book are not solely due to a wilful disregard for health but are the result of many factors including positive promotion by the advertising of products such as cigarettes and alcohol, of cultural and peer pressures, and of established social norms.

Heart disease

The disease which has greatly risen in incidence during the past 25 years is coronary heart disease, for which the UK still has the highest death rate in the world, with Northern Ireland and Scotland having higher death rates than England and Wales. While there has been a small reduction in mortality in recent years this must be placed against the background of our alarmingly high figures. The governments of the USA and Australia have introduced vigorous public education campaigns and policies which have resulted in substantially fewer deaths from heart disease. In Chapter 4 we will discuss heart disease and its prevention in greater detail.

Smoking

Of these harmful behaviours, smoking is the greatest single cause of disease and death. Cigarettes are advertised in magazines, newspapers, and at many sporting fixtures. Each packet has a statement that smoking cigarettes may result in ill-health, introduced only after many years of pressure being exerted on tobacco companies. Smoking causes lung cancer but it is less well-known by the public that it is a major cause of coronary heart disease, peptic ulcers, bronchitis, and other respiratory diseases. Of every 1000 young men who smoke cigarettes, statistics show that 6 will die in road accidents and 250 will die prematurely as a result of smoking. Chapter 7 discusses smoking and the ways in which the pharmacist can help smokers to quit.

Alcohol

The cost of alcohol has decreased in real terms during the last two decades. Between 1970 and 1976, the price of beer fell by 4 per cent, wine by 14 per cent and spirits by 21 per cent compared with the Retail Price Index. Average disposable income increased by 17 per cent in real terms over the same period, thus further decreasing the true cost of alcohol. The number of licensed premises has increased, including supermarkets and off-licences, and alcohol is heavily advertised (almost £200 millions are spent annually on its promotion). Alcohol intake is implicated in road accident deaths, in violence, in suicide rates, cirrhosis of the liver, and in admission to psychiatric hospitals. Chapter 8 considers the effects of alcohol on health and discusses the concept and practicalities of 'safe drinking' limits.

Nutrition

Our British diet now contains highly processed foods—more than ever before—and consumers often have little idea of what they are eating. Processing often removes natural fibres from foods and adds sugar, salt, and fats. Artificial flavourings and colourings make processed foods more palatable, and preservatives ensure they can be kept on the supermarket shelf for longer. Two major reports published in the 1980s, the NACNE (National Advisory Committee on Nutrition Education) and COMA (Committee on Medical Aspects of Food Policy) reports, agreed that the most significant way in which our diet should change for better health was to reduce the total amount of fat and, within this, to reduce the amount of saturated fat that we eat. The traditional British diet of 'chips with everything' and large quantities of fat is an effective way to achieve a heart attack at an early age.

Sugar

Sugar is inexpensive and therefore included in a range of foods, but the inadequate regulations on food labelling mean the manufacturer is required to state only that it is present, not its quantity. For example, a well-known brand of muesli (promoted as a 'health food') was identified by Caroline Walker in 1984 in her book *The food scandal* as containing 21 per cent sugar. While our sugar intake is now in comparative decline it is still a contributory factor to overweight and obesity (over half of the British population are overweight, and one in twelve men, one in eight women sufficiently so to be termed 'obese'). The addition of sugar accustoms people to its taste, and a 'sweet tooth' is established in infancy, where many proprietary baby drinks and foods have high sugar contents. For the manufacturer, the ability to add sugar means the cost of the product is reduced, sugar being cheaper than many other ingredients. Both the NACNE and COMA (*Diet and cardiovascular disease*) reports recommend a reduction in sugar consumption.

Salt

Salt is implicated in the incidence of hypertension and heart disease, and one half of all the salt we eat is in processed foods so that often we do not know when we are eating it.

Fibre

Fibre is removed from flour-based products such as bread, then salt and sugar are added. Lack of fibre is implicated as a causative factor in some cancers and bowel disease, and the NACNE and COMA reports were in agreement that our diet should contain more fibre. The amount of wholemeal bread now consumed is rising, although the average British intake of fibre is still well below the recommended levels.

The relationship between income and nutrition

Lower income groups spend a greater percentage of their disposable income but less in actual money on food than do those in higher income groups. In a diet that contains excessive quantities of sugars and fats, they are likely to eat less fresh fruit, green vegetables, and wholemeal bread and more white bread and sugar. Healthy eating changes have been shown by research to have occurred more quickly and to a greater extent in people of higher socioeconomic groups. The cost of many 'healthy' foods is often higher than the alternatives—for example, a wholemeal loaf costs more than the standard white version.

Differences in dietary and health choices, while undoubtedly linked to educational and cost considerations, are also likely to have cultural connotations. George Orwell noted in *The road to Wigan pier* that, if luxuries such as sweets and chocolates are the only ones which are affordable, then it is those which will be purchased. The same is true of alcohol, where price and affordability are major factors in increasing its consumption. The subject of healthy eating is discussed further in Chapter 9, where suggestions are given for the kinds of advice that pharmacists might offer.

Baby and child health

Young mothers and their children are a major client group in community pharmacies. Ensuring a high uptake of vaccination and immunization programmes is a vital element of public health, and pharmacists are well-placed to give clear information in this area. Chapter 10 discusses this and other aspects of child health.

Family planning and sexual health

A changing social climate and a reduction in the use of barrier contraceptive methods (until recently) has resulted in an increased incidence of sexually-transmitted diseases (STDs) of which AIDS is one. As the incidence of AIDS has risen and sexual behaviours have been modified, there has been an equivalent downturn in the incidences of other STDs such as gonorrhoea among homosexual men, although there is no such downturn for heterosexual men. Chapter 11 considers contraception and women's health, and the advice and information which pharmacists might offer.

Drug misuse

The number of intravenous drug users has risen, and it was estimated that in 1986 there were some 75 000–150 000 users of notifiable drugs in the UK. There were 14 785 'notified drug' users in the UK in 1989; thus the official figures are thought to underestimate the scale of the problem. While many will come to no harm through drug use, there is a serious risk that they will promote the spread of HIV infection by sharing needles and syringes. Chapter 12 addresses the role of the pharmacist in minimizing harm from drug misuse.

Four behaviours—smoking, diet, alcohol, and lack of exercise—are the most important areas where health promotion could have an effect, specifically on the incidence of coronary heart disease. The ways in which this health promotion is at present offered are examined next.

1.6.2 Strategies for change

In the preceding section we have shown the range of factors which combine to determine individual and community health, including economic status, physical environment, occupation and education, socioeconomic factors, and the provision and use of health services, as well as individual behaviour. All of these are potentially open to change through legislation and health promotion, ranging from action at community/societal level to that on an individual basis.

The community pharmacist has an important role to play in giving basic information to customers who seek it on, for example, vaccination programmes and infant feeding, taking part in specific activities such as anti-smoking campaigns, and as an intelligent and educated member of the community, able to explain current evidence on health matters. The Royal Pharmaceutical Society, too, is developing a higher profile in this field through the 'Pharmacy Healthcare' scheme and support for training initiatives. In Chapter 2 we will discuss the evolving role of the pharmacist in health promotion.

Government intervention

There are arguments for and against action at government as opposed to individual level for health. The importance of personal freedom and choice is sometimes cited as a reason not to pursue national policies of intervention. However, many health educators are agreed that without government intervention widespread change can be difficult, perhaps impossible, to achieve.

At the simplest level a government policy of increasing the tax levied on cigarettes and alcohol would produce a downturn in consumption. Statistics have shown conclusively that a rise in price of tobacco or alcohol products leads to a reduction in sales.

Recent years have seen cigarette advertising on television banned, but advertising in newspapers and magazines continues to be commonplace. Legislation to ban the advertising of cigarettes, such that cigarette advertisements did not subsequently reappear on television at sporting fixtures, would better enable consumers to make a free choice. The voluntary agreement on advertising involving tobacco companies does not ensure that tobacco sponsorship is not seen on television. Future generations are likely to note with disbelief that, even at the end of the twentieth century, advertising enticed young people to start smoking when it was known that cigarettes could only be harmful to health.

Currently, food manufacturers are legally required to provide only minimal information about their products on the product label. Some supermarket chains and individual companies have responded to consumer demand by providing more detailed nutrition information on the packaging of their foods. Nutrition information required by legislation and presented in simple terms would help consumers to identify the amounts of fat, sugar, and salt in the products they buy. The European Community is currently debating legal requirements for nutrition labelling, and the likely outcome is that food manufacturers will be forced to disclose more information on their labels.

Local and national pressure groups

Examples of local pressure in action are the demand for non-smoking areas in public places such as restaurants, cinemas, restaurants, and on public transport. National organizations such as ASH (Action on Smoking and Health) coordinate the activities of local groups and provide a lead and support for their activities. Using parliamentary lobbying and publicity campaigns, such groups have been very successful in raising public awareness and in achieving change.

1.7 Who offers health promotion?

The World Health Organization

The World Health Organization (WHO) defines health standards and conducts research into the links between health and factors such as environment, income, housing, and life stresses. It recognizes the need for local multi-disciplinary teams to examine not simply health facilities, but the opportunities for exercise, work, and recreation. The WHO policy document, *Health for all in the year 2000*, sets targets for the achievement of improved health by the promotion of lifestyles conducive to health, the reduction of preventable diseases, and the provision of healthcare accessible and acceptable to all.

Health Education Authority

The Health Education Authority (HEA) is funded by the Department of Health and acts as a separate health authority. In theory, it defines its own priorities, but critics argue that the government-funded HEA cannot pursue policies which are unpopular with its paymasters. An example of direct governmental intervention in the work of the Authority was the block placed on its proposed research on sexual behaviour in the context of the AIDS risk and the development of related health promotion programmes. This is one example of the way in which the ability of the Authority to act in an independent way in the interest of the nation's health has been brought into question.

The HEA and its predecessor, the Health Education Council, work by nationally-coordinated campaigns and by the publication and distribution of publicity and information materials on a wide range of health topics. Each year targets are set for health priorities and the Authority has been innovative in developing ways to monitor and evaluate health promotion programmes. It cannot, however, with much chance of success mount a political lobby against any particular government policy which legislates against health.

National pressure groups are not government-funded and may be a more potent political tool to effect change. Such groups (of which ASH, the British Heart Foundation, and MENCAP are probably the best-known) are extremely effective in acting as parliamentary lobbies to promote the interests of their members and to raise money for publicity, research, and educational materials.

District Health Authorities

District health promotion and health education services exist throughout the NHS, managed by a District Health Promotion Officer who has a staff establishment determined by the importance with which that health authority regards health promotion. There is, as yet, no strong coordination between the priorities set by the HEA and district health education services, who are better able to identify and respond to the particular needs of their health district.

We suggest that pharmacists who are interested in health promotion should establish working links with their local Health Education Promotion Officer, whose expertise and advice will be invaluable.

In this chapter we have examined definitions of health and its promotion. We have reviewed the changes in health which have occurred in the last century and the reasons for these changes. We have considered current health priorities and some possible strategies for change through a variety of means. In the next chapter we will look at the role of the pharmacist in health promotion.

2 The role of the pharmacist in health promotion

The prevention of ill-health is now seen as a priority for the health service. Within primary health care a new contract for general medical practitioners has emphasized screening and prevention activities. The pharmacist, too, is increasingly seen to have an important role in health promotion. Community pharmacies are visited by the healthy as well as by the sick, and the opportunities for health education inputs are great.

In the past, pharmacists have received little training in the area of health promotion, but the subject is gradually being introduced into undergraduate degree courses and now forms a significant proportion of continuing education programmes. In this chapter we will consider some of the events which have led to the recognition of the pharmacist as a health educator.

2.1 Development of the pharmacist's role in health promotion

During the last decade a number of projects have shown that the community pharmacist can play an effective part in health promotion activities. Some of the first pharmacy-based campaigns were conducted in the early 1980s and focused on a variety of areas, including smoking cessation, prevention of heart disease, blood pressure measurement, healthy eating, alcohol awareness, and safety of medicines. In anti-smoking campaigns, pharmacists have offered advice and counselling to clients on how to stop smoking and have provided written support material in the form of leaflets. One such study utilized a pharmacist facilitator who visited pharmacies to provide training and support for participating pharmacists and to coordinate and evaluate the project. The use of facilitators in health promotion is well-established in medical practice but the concept has yet to be extended into community pharmacy.

Blood pressure measurement in the pharmacy has provided the opportunity for pharmacists to offer advice on diet, smoking, and lifestyle, with referral to the general practitioner where necessary. A small percentage of community pharmacies offer a blood pressure measuring service. The monitoring of blood pressure has also allowed pharmacists to discuss anti-hypertensive therapy and patient compliance with their clients, adding another dimension to the health promotion role. In a study which examined pharmacist advice on general nutrition, the availability of leaflets on healthy eating provided a focus for pharmacists to offer advice about the dietary changes needed to promote health.

The first studies investigating cholesterol testing in community pharmacies were reported in 1989, showing how such testing could act as a focus for health education advice from the pharmacist about reducing the risk of coronary heart disease. Some pharmacies now offer a heart disease screening programme incorporating cholesterol and blood pressure measurement, where the client is also weighed and questioned about risk factors for heart disease. Appropriate advice on lifestyle change is then offered, with referral to the general practitioner for further investigation according to agreed protocols.

In the late 1980s the first syringe-needle exchange schemes were established in pharmacies in response to the growing risk of AIDS among intravenous drug misusers. Pharmacists participating in such schemes have offered free packs of syringes, needles, and condoms together with health education material and some have accepted used needles and syringes for disposal. A report by the Institute of Psychiatry published in 1990 showed the majority of pharmacists to be willing to sell or supply needles and syringes, to distribute information, and give advice to drug misusers, while just under half would be willing to accept used materials for disposal. The authors concluded that there was a role for community pharmacists in reducing the risk of AIDS to drug misusers by supplying clean equipment and giving information. They commented that appropriate training should be designed to prepare pharmacists for participation in schemes.

An important and influential group in pharmacists' involvement in health promotion has been the Pharmacy Advisory Group of the

Health Education Authority. Established in the early 1980s with the remit of advising the HEA on pharmaceutical matters, it now has a dual role and acts as a focus for health promotion activities with a pharmacy connection. A major research project to investigate the pharmacist's role in health promotion, *The pharmacist as a health educator* was completed in 1989 and concluded that, while the potential for the pharmacist in health promotion was high, there were a number of barriers to fuller participation. These included lack of training at undergraduate and postgraduate level, lack of remuneration, and lack of official recognition of health promotion activities.

2.1.1 The 'Healthcare in the High Street' scheme

Following a study of the potential role of the pharmacy as a site for the provision of health care information and advice, carried out by the Family Planning Association and Royal Pharmaceutical Society, the 'Healthcare in the High Street' scheme was launched in 1986. The scheme involved the first national distribution of health education leaflets through pharmacies. Jointly sponsored by the Royal Pharmaceutical Society, National Pharmaceutical Association, Health Education Authority, Scottish Health Education Group, and Family Planning Association, the new system distributed a display stand to each community pharmacy in England, Wales, Scotland, and Northern Ireland, followed by regular mailings of leaflets. Topics covered have included contraception, smoking cessation, food hygiene, prevention of heart disease and cancer, AIDS, drug abuse, and many others. Evaluations of the scheme found a consistently high utilization of the leaflet display stand (over 50 per cent) and that, while not always displayed in a prominent manner, leaflets were available in the majority of pharmacies visited (over 90 per cent). The willingness of pharmacists to participate in this unremunerated activity was thus demonstrated to be high and a telephone survey of community pharmacists showed a strong commitment to health education as part of their role.

'Healthcare in the High Street' did not receive government funding in its early years, and financial backing was sought from organizations such as the Health Education Authority and charities to print and distribute leaflets. Long-term planning was thus difficult and timing of supplies of leaflets and topics covered were necessarily sporadic, depending on the funds available. Many charitable organizations, including the Women's National Cancer Control Campaign and the British Heart Foundation, used the scheme to disseminate information. Response rates to coupons on the leaflets, where further information could be requested by the reader, were uniformly high and provided evidence that the leaflets were being read by those who took them from the pharmacy.

The renamed 'Pharmacy Healthcare' scheme continues the distribution of free leaflets on healthcare topics on a national basis. Central Government funding of £250 000 annually was announced in 1989 to secure the future of the project. With financial resources guaranteed, the selection of topics can become more structured and planned further in advance, allowing educational support for pharmacists to be provided in tandem. However, it must be noted that the sum made available by the government covers only the organization and running of the 'Pharmacy Healthcare' scheme and there is no element of remuneration for those pharmacists who take part. The Pharmaceutical Services Negotiating Committee (PSNC) is currently attempting to ensure that such payment is included in the NHS contract for community pharmacies, with support from the Royal Pharmaceutical Society of Great Britain (RPSGB).

Having reviewed the progress of the pharmacist's developing role in health promotion, we will now go on to look at the changes which are occurring in pharmacy practice and at how these changes might influence the further development of the pharmacist's role in health promotion.

2.1.2 The changing role of the pharmacist

Traditionally, the community pharmacist has been seen as a compounder and dispenser of medicines, and pharmacists' training has prepared them for this role. In fact, prior to the formation of the NHS pharmacists were more often a first port of call for those members of the public seeking advice about their ailments who could not afford medical advice from a doctor. The pharmacist's workload, too, has changed—in 1937 17 000 pharmacies dispensed 65 million prescriptions, but by 1980 the figures showed that 10 600 pharmacies were dispensing 360 million prescriptions each year. The reasons for this great change are complex and include the greater effectiveness of medicines, improved diagnostic facilities, greater life expectancy, and increased public expectations of health services. The result has been a trend for pharmacists to work in the dispensary dealing with prescriptions rather than in direct contact with members of the public.

Concurrent with the increasing proportion of the pharmacist's time spent on the dispensing of NHS prescriptions, one of the pharmacist's traditional roles, that of 'counter prescribing', has been reduced. Counter prescribing, or responding to symptoms, can be defined as the recommendation of over-the-counter medicines, advice to seek medical help when needed, and general advice to promote good health in response to a request for advice and treatment. Within the latter area falls a range of health education topics where there are opportunities for pharmacist intervention. These form the basis for the remainder of this book.

And what of the pharmacy customer or client? With the advent of the NHS the previous necessary emphasis on self-care and mainten-ance of good health was to some extent abandoned in favour of visits to the doctor's surgery. In the same era came the development of new medicines and the public perception became that these new drugs would provide 'a pill for every ill' and that the NHS would assume responsibility for everyone's health, leaving no need for self-care. These factors undermined the pharmacist's role as per-ceived by the public in advising about health matters. The situation has gradually altered over recent years, partly because of a growing awareness of individual behaviour as a cause of disease and a move towards self-care and greater individual responsibility for health, and partly because increasing prescription charges appear to have inhibited some patients from visiting the doctor. One outcome has been to move away from the 'a pill for every ill' philosophy towards seeking advice from health professionals to maintain health.

To summarize, the role of the community pharmacist is in the process of change, and we will look next at the key factors influenc-ing that change.

2.2 The impetus for change

There are three main sources providing impetus for change:

1. the profession itself:

2. consumer expectations and demands:

3. external bodies, including government.

2.2.1 The profession itself

All professions must respond to societal developments and changing consumer needs in order to survive. Should they fail to do so, consumers are likely to take their business elsewhere, or government may intervene to redefine professional practices. The *Nuffield report* was widely welcomed within pharmaceutical organizations and among pharmacists themselves. The concept of the extended role was embraced, although doubts were expressed about Nuffield's proposals for achieving this through 'relaxation' of supervision requirements for dispensing and sales of 'Pharmacy Only' medicines. Even before the Nuffield Inquiry, the advisory role of the community pharmacist was increasing in extent and importance.

In the early 1980s, the National Pharmaceutical Association (NPA) commissioned an advertising campaign to promote the advisory role of the community pharmacist, with the slogan 'Ask Your Pharmacist—You'll Be Taking Good Advice'. The campaign included magazine advertisements and limited television advertising and was shown by market research to have been very successful in increasing public awareness of the pharmacist's role, particularly in advice on minor illnesses and their treatment. Increased awareness of the role of the pharmacist in advising on prescription medicines and on health matters generally was also achieved, albeit to a lesser extent. The NPA campaign has continued since 1982, with a recent change of slogan to 'Ask An Expert—Ask Your Pharmacist'.

The campaign was appropriate for its time since the media were already beginning to inform the public about health in a way that encouraged the seeking of further information and advice. The advertising campaign for pharmacy gave consumers the impetus to seek this advice from the pharmacist. Anecdotal reports from community pharmacists are that the numbers of people requesting advice have greatly increased during the 1980s and there is a widely-held view that, while the NPA's advertising campaign has been partly responsible for this, the wider changes in consumer knowledge and demands have been of equal significance.

The Royal Pharmaceutical Society of Great Britain (RPSGB), as pharmacy's professional body, was supportive both of the Nuffield recommendations relating to health promotion and of those in the White Paper *Promoting better health*. The RPSGB continues to run the 'Pharmacy Healthcare' scheme and has been active in promoting the extension of payments to community pharmacists for services other than dispensing. The Society has also encouraged the inclusion of health promotion as a topic for continuing education programmes. While teaching on health promotion is not yet a requirement for all undergraduate pharmacy courses, the Pharmaceutical Society's working party on the teaching of social and behavioural sciences has recommended that it should be so, as has a Health Education Authority working group. Similar provision is already included in medical and nursing courses, where the fundamental importance of preventive measures and health promotion is now recognized and has become part of the syllabus.

Community pharmacists' negotiating body, the Pharmaceutical Services Negotiating Committee (PSNC), moved to a proactive stance in 1989 by conducting a feasibility study of cholesterol testing in community pharmacies. Results from the pilot study showed that such a service could successfully be provided in pharmacies and that consumer demand was high. Local Pharmaceutical Committees have initiated other projects which extend the role of the community pharmacist, including asthma screening (with sponsorship from the pharmaceutical industry) and blood pressure measurement. PSNC are now pressing for remuneration for these and other services.

2.2.2 Consumer expectations and demands

The growth of the consumer movement in recent years has led to many changes in our society, including the legislation controlling consumer rights and choices and accountability for proffered services. Consumer demand has led to an explosion of information on a wide range of topics including health; indeed the passing of the Freedom of Information Act in the USA was consumer-driven. Consumer lobbying has been a powerful influence in some areas of food manufacture involving pharmacy practice, leading, for example, to the reduction or removal of sugar from some baby foods, clearer labelling of food additives and preservatives, and their removal from many products. Again, commercial interests have responded more quickly than the legislators—for example, the Boots company now advertises all the baby foods they manufacture as being free from additives and preservatives.

To illustrate the changes that have taken place in attitudes to information provision which have impinged on pharmacy practice, it is of note that as recently as 20 years ago the name of the drug or medicine dispensed was not included on the dispensed medicine label. The rationale for this policy was that patients did not need to know the name of their medicine. The situation has changed to the extent that there is currently a consumer-led movement to allow patients access to general practitioner and hospital medical records and all details of their medical history.

The public's demand for knowledge brings into sharp focus the dilemma of health professionals such as pharmacists and doctors, whose knowledge base has previously not been accessible to, or understood by, their clients. Knowledge has long been a source of power for professional groups, and any advance by consumers into the health knowledge base has resulted in expressed concern by health professionals that the lay person's lack of detailed under-standing may lead to unfounded fears. In reality, the concern being expressed was that professional groups regard any narrowing of the gulf in knowledge between health professional and client as a threat to their professional status.

The European Community's series of directives on medicines addresses the area of patient information and is likely to require that patient information leaflets be issued with all medicines, giving details that include side-effects and their incidence. Thus, decisions about information-giving will no longer be inherently within the control of health professionals.

The media and health consumerism

The role of the media has been crucial in raising the level of public awareness and education about health. In particular, television programmes such as *Horizon* and *World in Action* have accepted the consumer's right to be informed on matters of concern, includ-ing health. In some cases the media have exposed situations where parliamentary lobbies and vested interests had previously acted to limit public availability of information. Examples of such reporting include research evidence linking diet to health—specifically the harmful effects of diets high in dairy products and saturated fats. More recently, television programmes have provoked extensive public discussion and concern about the potential problems caused by *Salmonella* in eggs, *Listeria* in foods, and the possible transmission of bovine spongiform encephalopathy (BSE) from animals to humans. Such programmes have disseminated research findings to a mass audience. Television programmes on health topics are capable of offering information at an extremely high and detailed level. Other media—for example, national newspapers and women's magazines—now routinely feature items on health matters.

The 'quality' newspapers generally feature accurate and well-researched features, but for some newspapers health reporting is largely on topics which are thought likely to increase newspaper sales, that is sensational articles about areas of concern—for example, drug side-effects—without reminding readers of the possible benefits of the treatment concerned. It can also be argued that newspapers and other publications which rely on sponsorship and advertising are unlikely to publicize aspects of health education which are against the interests of their advertisers, so that a newspaper in which cigarettes are heavily advertised, for example, may be unlikely to publicize the harmful effects of smoking.

The accuracy of the information presented is sometimes doubtful, leading to apparent conflicts of information and health messages. Members of the public are not always in a position to separate truthful from incorrect information, and it is important that professional bodies act to point out inaccuracies and that health professionals advise their clients accordingly.

A well-informed public requires health professionals to update their own knowledge base, since their clients may be knowledgeable about their disease and its treatment. For example, articles and television programmes about the risks and benefits of drug therapy have led to a recognition among consumers that there are health choices and that an informed choice can be made about whether or not to have a particular treatment. Surgeons are now required to explain the potential benefits and risks of surgical procedures to patients. Consumers are more likely to seek further information from health professionals such as pharmacists, who are readily accessible.

The 'Health industry'

The increased public awareness of the fact that leading a healthier lifestyle will maintain good health has led to the development of a 'health industry', for example 'health food' shops, creating the perception that anything bought there will lead to good health. The sales of vitamins and dietary supplements, 'alternative' medicines, and 'health foods' from such outlets have effectively challenged the pharmacist's advisory role on health matters, since assistants in health food stores have been shown to offer advice and to respond to requests for advice about their companies' products. The quality of advice given in such cases is not established.

Another commercial response to increased public interest in health matters has been that of supermarket chains such as Tesco in their commendable aim to offer detailed nutritional advice and information to their customers, including food labelling which goes far beyond current legislative requirements. The St Ivel company modified its product range to include low-fat alternatives to its dairy products, an approach which has since been followed by other companies. The Boots company offers information leaflets on nutrition in their pharmacies and a computerized nutritional analysis of customers' diets is offered in some stores.

Consumers and health professionals

What consumers want from health professionals is information about their medicines and about their illnesses. Research shows that they would like health professionals to spend more time talking to them. A recent Consumers Association study examined what patients wanted from their GP and found that over 80 per cent of respondents wished to have more information and explanation about their disease and its drug treatment. In short, they wanted their doctor to spend more time talking to them about their health. Market research involving pharmacy customers has shown that, where the pharmacist gives information and is prepared to spend time at the counter, consumers welcome this. Studies on patient information leaflets demonstrated that patients appreciated them, that they read the information contained in the leaflets, and were not put off their drug therapy by being told about common side-effects.

Consumers' perception of pharmacists is often that they are relatively inaccessible and too busy in the dispensary. Market research shows that, whilst the pharmacist's advice is willingly given, consumers say that the consultation often had to be sought or requested by the customer rather than being volunteered by the pharmacist. Pharmacists' perceptions, on the other hand, are that they are readily accessible and available to their customers. The difference is wide.

2.2.3 External bodies, including government

During the last decade pharmacy has been subject to intense scrutiny from outside the profession as part of a governmental process of examining the role of all professions and their monopoly of practice. The thrust of government action has been to remove restrictive practices where these were not considered justifiable. Outcomes of this policy have included the removal of solicitors' monopoly on conveyancing and approval being given for spectacles to be sold from any commercial outlet. Against this background, then, pharmacy became the subject of an inquiry into its practice and future role.

In 1981 the then Minister of Health, Gerard Vaughan, stated in his opening address at the British Pharmaceutical Conference that, whilst he could clearly see a future for hospital and industrial pharmacists, there was no identified role for the community pharmacist. Pharmacists, he said, enjoyed the public's trust but were unable to make full use of their skills. His and similar concerns led to the setting-up of the Nuffield Inquiry in October 1983 with a brief to examine all aspects of pharmacy from undergraduate education to professional practice, to make recommendations for the future, and in particular to see how the profession of pharmacy could meet the needs of its consumers.

The *Nuffield report* was published in 1986, and its fundamental thrust for community pharmacy was that pharmacists must move towards an extended advisory role and away from a purely technical dispensing function. Within the extended role, health promotion was clearly identified by the Nuffield Inquiry as an area in which pharmacists should become more greatly involved, reflected in the statement that 'there is a role for pharmacists in health education in cooperation with other health professionals'.

Several of the recommendations from the *Nuffield report* featured in the White Paper *Promoting better health*, published in November 1987, which outlined future strategy and policy for primary healthcare. Again, health promotion was clearly identified as an important area for development in community pharmacy. *Promoting better health* contained a statement of intent to provide core funding for the provision of health education materials in community pharmacies. This promise was fulfilled in April 1989, when Kenneth Clarke, the then Secretary of State for Health, announced funding of £250 000 annually for the development of the 'Health in the High Street' information scheme and other facets of health promotion in pharmacy.

Of fundamental importance for pharmacy within *Promoting better health* was the statement of intent to begin to move remuneration for community pharmacy away from the basis of dispensing prescriptions and towards the provision of other services, as Nuffield had recommended. The first such services were the provision of pharmaceutical services to residential homes and the establishment and keeping of patient medication records for elderly and confused patients. The Minister for Health has announced that legislative change will allow further developments of this type by widening the definition of 'pharmaceutical services' which can be remunerated from the NHS. The NHS and Community Care Bill carried an amendment to this end.

Having considered key influences on pharmacy practice, we will now turn to the pharmacy as a setting for health promotion activities. For pharmacists who wish to develop their role in this area, an awareness of strengths and weaknesses of pharmacy-based health promotion is essential.

2.3 Advantages and disadvantages of health promotion activities in the pharmacy

2.3.1 The consumer viewpoint

A fundamental strength of community pharmacies is that they are outside the formal referral system of the NHS, in contrast to medical services, and members of the public can visit a pharmacy anonymously. Advice can be sought from any pharmacist the person chooses and a 'second opinion' obtained from a different pharmacy if desired. No appointment is needed to speak to a pharmacist and the consumer is under no obligation to accept or act on the advice offered. A pharmacist can be readily selected on the basis of age or gender, not always the case in medical practice.

Pharmacies are readily accessible as part of the everyday shopping environment, and each has an informed advisor whose advice is free. Research has shown that the pharmacist's advice is well-respected by consumers and that the percentage of the public who are prepared to seek that advice continues to increase. A consultation may end in one of three ways—with referral to the general practitioner, recommendation of an over-the-counter medicine or advice only, or a mixture of these elements.

The consumer can choose which pharmacy to visit, and whilst the majority of patients usually elect to have their prescriptions dispensed at the same pharmacy, this may not be so for other services—for example, cholesterol testing. This facility to choose a pharmacy is of critical importance in potentially sensitive areas such as pregnancy testing, where a consumer may not want the test to be carried out at their local pharmacy.

The pharmacist's code of ethics requires him to maintain absolute confidentiality on patient information, and this is of obvious benefit to consumers who may wish to discuss sensitive and private issues with the pharmacist. Members of the public may be unaware of the ethical requirement for confidentiality and wider publicity for its existence might be helpful.

The lack of privacy in community pharmacies is a disadvantage, and over half the pharmacy customers interviewed in market research considered that their regular pharmacy lacked sufficient privacy to discuss confidential subjects. However, some customers prefer the type of 'open chat' which can be held in the pharmacy and are unconcerned about the lack of more private consultation facilities. We shall discuss the subject of privacy in community pharmacies in the next chapter.

There is potential tension between the professional role of a pharmacist as a health professional and the commercial role in operating a business, and a high proportion of customers who ask for advice about symptoms are sold an over-the-counter medicine, while some 10–20 per cent are referred to their doctor without any such sale being made. Sociologists have found that a high level of professionalism exists alongside a high level of business awareness for many pharmacists. This is exemplified by a community pharmacist's statement that:

> The professional decision is often a good commercial decision. There's not as much conflict long-term as you would think. At that moment you lose out commercially. But long-term your standing with the public is a very good commercial asset . . . when you've got a regular clientele they get to know your honesty's valuable.

Client expectations in a commercial environment such as a pharmacy are often to purchase a medicine, and many pharmacy customers go to the pharmacy with the intention of doing so. The dilemma of whether to provide patients with what they ask for is not unique to pharmacy, and the example of the issue of prescriptions to over three-quarters of GPs' patients is often cited as a result of patient demand rather than best medical practice.

Some groups—that is, those who are exempt from prescription charges (elderly people, the unemployed)—may believe that they will have to buy a product if they ask a pharmacist for advice. This belief may, in some cases, discourage the seeking of advice.

Consumers have little awareness that pharmacists know about health promotion, which may seem to them far removed from pharmacists' well-known or accepted knowledge base of medicines and drugs. Research conducted by the Consumers' Association and presented in evidence to the Nuffield Inquiry showed that consumers were reluctant to ask pharmacists about general health matters, or to seek screening tests from pharmacies. However, when such tests are offered in pharmacies the demand is high, and with the increasing availability of screening tests in pharmacies—for example, for high blood pressure and serum cholesterol—public awareness of the pharmacist's ability to advise on health promotion should be enhanced.

To customers, the pharmacy must seem a very busy place where the pharmacist has little time to do anything other than make up prescriptions in the dispensary. Thus they feel they will be interrupting the pharmacist's work by requesting advice and there is research evidence showing that 80 per cent of requests from consumers are dealt with, at least initially, by counter assistants. This has two results: the first is a public perception that the level of advice available is low and that it may come only from counter assistants;

the second is that, in order to ask for the pharmacist's advice, the assistant's advice will be seen to be rejected.

2.3.2 The pharmacist's viewpoint

The first advantage is that involvement in health promotion activities more clearly demonstrates that the pharmacist is a member of the primary healthcare team—that is, dealing in the community with aspects of lifestyle and behaviour which, left unaltered, would lead to the development of health problems. If screening programmes are offered in the pharmacy, the referral policies and protocols will mean that the pharmacist has a greater contact with local medical practitioners and other members of the healthcare team. With this increased contact, particularly with medical practitioners, the pharmacist's image and status will be enhanced, since a non-commercial activity is involved. At the same time pharmacists will be demonstrating their healthcare knowledge base. In addition to this change in image as seen by medical practitioners, the consumer's image of the pharmacist should also be enhanced—that is, the pharmacist will come to be seen as an expert in healthcare rather than simply as a dispenser of medicines.

Involvement in health promotion activities utilizes a greater amount of the pharmacist's health knowledge base and training. It also involves the pharmacist in the development of professional practice in line with current thinking. One potential commercial benefit of operating a screening programme from a pharmacy is that more customers will visit the shop. If the range of subjects on which the pharmacist's customers perceive he can give advice is wide, then that advice is likely to be sought more often and will involve yet more visits to the pharmacy. Furthermore, each time effective advice is given the image of the pharmacist as a giver of good advice is reinforced in the customer's mind, leading to repeat visits and customer loyalty.

The greater involvement of the pharmacist in discussions with customers will have the additional benefit of providing continual training for counter assistants (who can offer simple advice themselves and will better recognize when the pharmacist needs to be involved). It will also lead to a greater recognition of the pharmacist's knowledge. Counter assistants' perceptions of pharmacists are also that they are busy people, and an assistant may be unwilling to interrupt a pharmacist, so a demonstrated willingness on the pharmacist's part to give advice will result in more frequent referrals.

Participation in health promotion campaigns and activities, and their advertisement within the pharmacy, leads to requests for information from other members of the healthcare team such as district nurses and health visitors, and members of the public such as teachers may request that the pharmacist gives a talk at the local school on a health topic. Thus, among other professionals there is heightened awareness of what the pharmacist is able to do.

The pharmacist's time, or lack of it, is a potential disadvantage in involvement in health promotion activities both from the point of view of requests for advice and those occasions where opportunistic advice could be given. These are most likely to occur when the shop is at its busiest—at peak prescription-dispensing times—and customers take the opportunity to ask for information and advice. Thus, the availability of short, well-structured advice models could help pharmacists to make the best use of a limited amount of time, and the use of trained dispensing technicians, to whom the bulk of prescription-dispensing can be delegated, will free the pharmacist's time. For screening tests, the problem of the pharmacist's time can be overcome by using appointment systems, and in some cases another strategy might be the employment of a second pharmacist on a part-time basis.

Pharmacists' traditional undergraduate training has not included health promotion, communication skills, and the social background to health issues. Pharmacists have therefore not been in the best position from which to offer advice. Changes in the undergraduate syllabus will alleviate this problem for new undergraduates, but for those pharmacists who are already registered continuing education programmes will be required to ensure familiarity with these subjects as well as targeted articles in the pharmaceutical press.

The potential costs of converting parts of the pharmacy to provide a consulting room or a consultation area are high and there is currently no government reimbursement for such alterations. The pharmacist currently receives no payment for the advice given, particularly since the demise of the cost-plus contract, before which an element of the remuneration system reimbursed pharmacists for time spent in advice relating to NHS matters. The use of remuneration systems to effect changes in the practices of health professionals can be an effective means of achieving objectives. For example, the new general practitioner contract, with its targets for immunization and targeted payments for health promotion activities, is likely to increase the percentage of the target groups reached.

Linked to the question of payment for services in the case of health promotion advice is the fact that the pharmacist, when not selling a product, has no means of receiving payment for time spent. In the world of small businesses, where time necessarily means money, pharmacists are unlikely to change their practices substantially unless such disincentives are removed. However, in health promotion research projects based in pharmacies, pharmacists have taken the view that the high level of uptake and appreciation by their customers of the service being offered is likely to have enhanced customer loyalty, and thus the pharmacist may regard the time spent as an investment for future return.

2.4 Future development of health promotion in the pharmacy

Appropriate knowledge and skills in health promotion are essential for the underpinning of pharmacist involvement. With the introduction of core teaching in pharmacy undergraduate courses on health promotion, followed by provision in continuing education programmes, further role development will be possible.

The potential for community pharmacists to be paid for services other than NHS dispensing will be a key factor in the development of health promotion services. The Pharmaceutical Services Negotiating Committee has already proposed that remuneration should be provided for the display of health education materials and for the provision of a consultation room or area. Suggestions that screening tests should be paid for through the NHS contract have been made and are being pursued. The most difficult health promotion service to quantify is the giving of advice by the pharmacist, because of the problems inherent in defining parameters such as quality and standards for such a service. Nevertheless, the future for an appropriately-remunerated service looks hopeful.

In this chapter we have examined the changing role of the community pharmacist and some of the pressures for change, both from within and outside the profession. The advantages and draw-backs of providing health promotion through pharmacies have been explored from the consumer's and the pharmacist's viewpoint. The development of the community pharmacist's role in health promotion has been briefly reviewed and the prospects for further development considered. In the next chapter we will look at the importance of communication skills in the practice of health promotion in a pharmacy context.

3 Communication in health promotion

The psychology of human behaviour, and of means by which it might be altered, is complex. In order to give effective advice on health promotion, the pharmacist must understand that even behaviours which are known to create a risk to health can be difficult to change. At the core of the required interpersonal skills for pharmacists are the ability to advise, educate, influence, and persuade customers to adopt healthier lifestyles. In this chapter we will discuss the importance of effective interpersonal skills in the pharmacy, and means by which such skills may be developed. Necessary changes in the pharmacy environment to facilitate better communication are proposed.

3.1 The challenge — what are the potential difficulties in communication?

3.1.1 Changing behaviour and lifestyle

The area of health promotion contains many apparent contradictions. For example, large numbers of the population understand that smoking and inappropriate diet can lead to coronary heart disease, yet many people continue to smoke and to consume foods which are not the most healthy. In order for the pharmacist to offer advice about health promotion which has any chance of being accepted, it is essential to have an understanding of some of the reasons underlying continued behaviours which constitute a risk to health.

Educational, social, and cultural background all have a major part to play in determining a person's response to ill-health and attitude towards maintaining good health. Underlying attitudes determine the extent to which particular issues are addressed or avoided. These attitudes and beliefs may or may not be openly acknowledged or expressed by pharmacy customers.

Attitudes to food, for example, are formed early in life, and research has shown that it is easier to influence the diet of younger than older children. Food preferences are strongly influenced by the social and environmental context in which food is offered to children. Pairing nutritious foods such as fresh vegetables with parental attention resulted in these foods becoming more attractive to children in one study, illustrating the interlinking of foods and emotional relationships. The formation of attitudes and behaviour towards food in the early years helps to explain the findings from numerous studies, that achieving long-term change in eating patterns is difficult.

Cigarette smoking, too, is a behaviour with social and emotional overtones. People who start to smoke as part of a peer group may come to associate smoking with friendliness, a feeling of 'belonging', and enjoyment. These underlying attitudes are attacked in campaigns which emphasize the antisocial nature and dirtiness of smoking.

The ability of the pharmacist to influence the customer's behaviour is likely itself to be affected by the pharmacist's own attitudes and beliefs. Positive attitudes towards the prevention of ill-health are fundamental and health professionals must maintain a non-judgemental approach if their advice is to be accepted.

Various sociological models have been proposed to try to explain people's behaviour in relation to health. The 'Health Belief' model is one of the most widely known and it suggests that actions taken to maintain health, or in response to ill-health, are related to the perceived seriousness and risks involved and the perceived benefits of taking the particular course of action or treatment being offered. A variety of factors influence health behaviour and one key skill for the pharmacist might be defined as 'persuading' to influence behaviour.

Research has shown that people have widely varying concepts of what constitutes health and of the nature of health risks. A recent study showed that, of 100 men under the age of 60 who had had a heart attack, 85 smoked but only one in three believed that smoking had anything to do with their heart attack. Many of these men had seen or heard information which suggested that smoking and heart disease were linked, but their health belief was that this was not the case. Instead, many believed that stress was the most important factor in the development of their condition.

People make health choices by making their own estimate of the likely physical and emotional consequences of their actions. This estimate may be favourable or unfavourable, and behaviour is maintained or altered depending on the person's subjective estimate of the likely outcomes. Attitudes and beliefs about health are developed by the social and political context in which they arise, and by a process of social learning.

Health education is based on the premise that beliefs and attitudes are malleable and can be changed by persuasion and information. The assumption is that changes in attitudes and beliefs will lead to changes in behaviour.

So there are two aspects, *beliefs* and *evaluation*. To take smoking as an example, a smoker may accept that they will have an increased risk of dying prematurely from heart disease or lung cancer. On the other hand, the immediate value of smoking as a coping strategy in a difficult life is one factor which will affect the decision to stop, because the person's belief about stopping smoking may be that they will be unable to cope with everyday life. The long-term benefits of smoking, i.e. living longer, may not be attractive to someone whose life is unhappy and poor. The smoker may also believe that the health damage has already been done and that there is therefore no benefit to be gained by stopping.

Thus, patients do not always follow patterns of behaviour and life-style which are the most conducive to good health, even when information is available to them. There are two major issues in health promotion activity for the pharmacist from the point of view of advice-giving: the educational aspect, which informs patients, and the pharmacist's interpersonal skills in influencing and persuading the individual to modify their lifestyle.

3.1.2 The influence of personal factors

Personal factors relating to both pharmacist and customer/client impinge on the communication process and their importance must be acknowledged.

The **pharmacist's** own attitudes, beliefs, values, and standards can lead to judgements being made about the worth, intelligence, and genuineness of the client. Health professionals must recognize that their customers' or patients' knowledge and beliefs have emerged from their life experience, whereas those of health professionals have been developed, extended, and modified by professional education and training. It is essential that pharmacists try to accept and understand their patients' point of view, not make value judgements.

Appearance and stereotypes influence communication; a classic example is where some pharmacists make incorrect assumptions— such as, when speaking to elderly people, conversing in a loud voice and using childishly simple language. 'Ageism' is unfortunately common throughout our society, and the assumption that becoming deaf and rather stupid are natural accompaniments of growing old is obviously incorrect.

Another typical pharmacy example occurs when the scruffily-dressed young man or woman asks to buy a medicine known to be subject to abuse, such as codeine linctus. Value judgements are often made on the basis of appearance, and while many pharmacists would automatically be suspicious of such a customer, the same request from a smartly-dressed middle-aged man might initially provoke fewer suspicions.

Stereotypes which relate intelligence and need for information to socioeconomic status are also prevalent. Some pharmacists assume that, because their practice is in a deprived area, their customers and patients are less intelligent and neither want nor need additional information. Customers from more affluent areas may be perceived as demanding more attention and having a greater ability to understand what they are told. It is better to make decisions about information and advice-giving on an individual basis.

Particular styles of dress and appearance lead to the formation of value judgements on the pharmacist's part and personal prejudices may then act as a barrier to communication. As pharmacists we must be aware of these opinions and prejudices and must learn to attempt not to make assumptions based on first impressions.

The speed at which the pharmacist speaks is of great importance. Pharmacists are often working under intense pressure, especially when a number of prescriptions are waiting to be dispensed. However, research has shown that, when under such pressure, pharmacists are likely to speak very fast in giving information and explanations, and that their customers consequently remembered little of what they had been told. A conscious effort to speak slowly and clearly is thus required.

For the **patient**, attitudes and beliefs about health and the pharmacist as a credible source of information and advice will affect the extent to which that advice is believed and accepted. Gender and age are important; for example, an elderly patient may not accept that a young pharmacist has sufficient knowledge or experience to be able to offer advice. Cross-gender communication may act as a barrier to communication if, for example, an elderly male is experiencing urinary problems but is reluctant to talk to a female pharmacist because of his belief that she 'will not understand' the problem and of his embarrassment at having to explain his symptoms. The 'problems' in such cases are often perceived rather than actual.

3.1.3 Language and jargon

There are many ways in which language can influence the communication process; some are listed below.

- Foreign language/language barrier

- Accent

- Regional dialect

- Regional phrases and terms

- Limit of vocabulary

- Use of jargon

The vocabulary and language used by the pharmacist is a major influence on the customer's understanding. During their training every health professional learns the jargon associated with their professional group. It then becomes all too easy to speak in terms which the layman cannot understand. The vocabulary range of most members of the public is very limited and, generally speaking, the higher the educational level, the wider the vocabulary. Pharmacists need to make a constant effort to speak in simple terms and to avoid jargon and technical terms wherever possible. Examples overheard by the authors include:

1. A young hospital pharmacist had just dispensed a prescription for a young child for sustained release aminophylline capsules.

> Pharmacist: So it's one capsule morning and night.
> Mother: She's only 7, she'll never be able to swallow these. Can I tip the powder into some jam?
> Pharmacist: Well the thing is, they're sustained release.
> Mother (completely ignoring the pharmacist's comment): But can I tip them out on to some jam so she can swallow it?

2. Experienced community pharmacist responding to a request for information about an over-the-counter medicine.

> Customer: What about those Nurofen tablets then—how do they work?
> Pharmacist: It's a non-steroidal anti-inflammatory.
> Customer (bewildered): Oh, I see.

Such examples are common and represent, not an attempt to 'blind the patient with science', but the pharmacist's forgetting that his customers do not have the same vocabulary as he does. Sometimes the use of a technical term is unavoidable, and if that is the case the term should be introduced and then explained.

The pharmacist may even speak a different language from his customers. Research in pharmacies in inner-city Birmingham with a high proportion of Asian customers showed a significant number of pharmacies where neither the pharmacist nor any member of staff spoke the language in question. This is increasingly recognized as a potential problem and it is possible that medicine labels in different languages giving common instructions may soon be available. For many pharmacies, if the pharmacist does not speak the language, employment of a staff member who does can go some way to improving things. Some pharmacists have learned how to pronounce specific instructions in other languages. This approach was adopted at some Bradford and Birmingham hospitals. The problem of course is that, should the patient then ask questions, the pharmacist is unable to respond.

There is a myth among health professionals that people from ethnic minorities are largely illiterate. Such thinking is based on the situation that ruled many years ago with first-generation immigrants. More recent research has shown that around one in five Asian patients are unable to read English or their own language. The remaining 80 per cent could read one or both, showing that the production of leaflets and labels could be valuable. As the number of first-generation immigrants declines and more family members learn to speak and read English, the problem will become less acute.

In the meantime the Health Education Authority produces a range of leaflets on topics such as health in pregnancy, infant feeding, and nutrition. Locally-produced leaflets may be available from your District Health Promotion Unit. Pharmacists who are considering preparing labels or leaflets in other languages should be aware that a direct translation is not always appropriate, since the meaning and sense of statements can be lost. Any such material should be carefully piloted via local community groups.

For pharmacists who work in areas with a high proportion of customers from ethnic minorities, contact with the local Health Promotion Unit can identify the languages most commonly spoken. For one Birmingham district these were Urdu and Punjabi—but, for other areas, different Asian languages, Polish, or Chinese may predominate, for example. Having identified the language, the pharmacist may then obtain stocks of leaflets from the sources identified above.

3.1.4 Situational factors—the pharmacy environment

The pharmacy itself can form a barrier to effective communication. Pharmacies are public and often busy places where it can be difficult to hold a private conversation. We have considered the question of privacy and we can identify here other elements in the pharmacy which may preclude good communication. The shop may be noisy, busy, and a place where conversations may easily be overheard. The traditional medicines counter itself acts as a physical barrier to communication and creates distance between pharmacist and patient.

The traditional layout of the pharmacy generally has its main points of activity located around the dispensary reception area and the medicines counter. For many smaller pharmacies these two may be the same. In a typical pharmacy there will be several patients waiting for their prescriptions to be dispensed, other shoppers browsing and looking at merchandise, while others are paying for their purchases or asking about particular items. There is thus an audience for any conversation which might take place.

3.1.5 Privacy and confidentiality

While pharmacists may be happy to discuss what to them are everyday subjects related to health, their customers may prefer a more private atmosphere. Indeed, research shows that over half of pharmacy customers say that sometimes they have not sought advice about a particular subject in a pharmacy because of the lack of privacy. There are numerous subject areas which are potentially sensitive—among the most obvious are symptoms which patients might be embarrassed to talk about, such as haemorrhoids, diarrhoea, and constipation, the communication of results of pregnancy and other tests, and advice on topics such as family planning.

Later in this chapter we will discuss ways in which the pharmacy environment needs to change to facilitate more privacy.

3.2 Which communication skills are required?

The elements of good communication have been described extensively by other authors. In this section we will briefly comment on the essential features of interpersonal communication and their relevance to pharmacy practice and health promotion. Written communication in the form of patient leaflets is increasingly recognized as a means of reinforcing verbal advice and is also considered. A list of further reading on the subject of communication can be found at the end of the chapter.

Communication should be a two-way process between pharmacist and patient or client. One of the myths about communication is that 'good communicators are born, not made'. In fact this is not true, and an awareness of the rudiments of the skills needed, preferably combined with communication skills training and followed by reflection on the pharmacist's own practice, can produce substantial improvements in an individual's ability to communicate. Training courses are available in most parts of the UK and are organized by Local Course Organizers for pharmacists. We will now go on to consider the key factors about the pharmacy environment and the pharmacist which influence communication.

3.2.1 Advice-giving and counselling

Many pharmacists consider these terms to be synonymous and often refer to 'patient counselling'. In fact they describe quite different activities and it is important to understand their differentiating features. **Counselling** has been defined as 'the means by which one person helps another to clarify their life situation and to decide upon further lines of action', and its aim is 'to give the client an opportunity to explore, discover, and clarify ways of living more resourcefully and towards greater well-being'. Counselling seeks to enable the patient or client to decide on a particular course of action and to see it through. Key skills in counselling include listening and empathy.

In **advice-giving**, information is passed from the health professional to the client in a two-way exchange and the client or patient should play an active part in the consultation. Here, the pharmacist is offering information and advice and educating the customer or patient.

In **instruction**, the input tends to be information passed from pharmacist to patient—in effect the pharmacist directs the patient as to which action to take. An example of such instruction is where the pharmacist reinforces the instructions on a medicine label: 'Take this medicine three times a day after food.' Good instruction should be a two-way process, with the pharmacist inviting feedback from the customer.

Counselling skills can be separated into two distinct areas: non-verbal and verbal. The first embraces the skills of listening and attending, the second those of verbal interventions. Counselling takes place in a variety of situations, many of which are relevant to health, including drug-abuse and alcohol problems and pregnancy termination (the latter including genetic counselling where genetic defects may be or have been identified). The area of HIV testing is currently one of great concern, and counselling before such a test is now known to be essential in order that the patient understands the consequences of the result they are about to obtain—that is to say, if a positive result is obtained, currently there is little that can be offered in the way of treatment or an improved prognosis.

To demonstrate the extent to which counselling involves discussion about emotions and feelings, and the negotiation of a course of action which is acceptable to the patient or client, consider the following list which describes the changes that may take place after counselling. These personal changes are based on observation and evaluation of clients who have gone through the counselling process.

- The person comes to see himself differently
- He accepts himself and his feelings more fully
- He becomes more confident and self-directing
- He becomes more flexible, less rigid, in his perceptions
- He behaves in a more mature fashion
- He becomes more acceptant of others
- He changes his basic personality characteristics in constructive ways

(Adapted from Rogers 1967)

These features demonstrate that counselling may be a lengthy process, involving significant discussion. Pharmacists will be familiar with the Alcoholics Anonymous organization and with community organizations where drug misusers are counselled, as examples of health-related counselling.

We suggest that, generally, counselling is *not* what takes place in community pharmacies and that pharmacists are involved in the giving of information and advice which suggests or directs the course of action the patient should take and where the focus is health. The advice-giving which pharmacists undertake in their everyday practice is clearly more appropriate to the community pharmacy setting. While pharmacists may sometimes use the skills of counselling, they are largely concerned with giving information to clients and trying to ensure that this information is understood.

Advice-giving relating to prescription medicines will be generated in two types of situation: firstly, the pharmacist may volunteer information and advice in relation to a prescription; or secondly, the pharmacist's advice will be prompted by a request from the patient for information. Here, explaining skills are vital so that the patient understands the information given. In responding to symptoms, the pharmacist's advice relates to a request from the patient, and here the skills of questioning assume great importance in determining possible causes of the problem and formulating appropriate advice. Opportunistic health promotion advice can be offered in relation to prescription medicines and in response to symptoms. Here, the patient or client has not directly asked the pharmacist for such advice but the opportunity arises through the symptom or medicine being discussed. For example, in questioning a patient about a cough the pharmacist may find that the person is a heavy smoker; or, in discussing a baby's nappy rash with the mother, he may be able to give much-needed advice on nappy changing and skin care to prevent recurrence.

3.2.2 Listening

'Being a good listener' is as much a skill as a natural state. The verbal and non-verbal features which make a speaker recognize whether or not he is being listened to can be learned by the pharmacist. **Non-verbal** signs, including establishing and maintaining eye contact, smiling, nodding, and the use of posture (in leaning towards the patient) all signify that the listener is paying attention. Conversely, avoiding eye contact, a bored or inattentive expression or behaviours, or a posture which leans away from the patient all suggest that the listener is not paying attention. **Verbal** signs can indicate that careful listening is going on and these include occasional comments which do not interrupt the flow of conversation from the speaker. Thus the nodding of the head can be supplemented by brief verbal contributions such as 'Yes' or 'Ah-ha'. Questions and comments can also be used to show interest, create empathy, and demonstrate listening, examples being 'Did he?', 'Really?', and exclamations such as 'Oh, no!', 'How terrible/ wonderful!', and so on.

Sometimes it is difficult not to interrupt what a patient is saying— for example, in responding to symptoms, if the pharmacist thinks he has identified the cause of the problem or if the customer makes a factually incorrect statement or one with which the pharmacist strongly disagrees. However, in good communication the listener will rarely interrupt the speaker. In practice, everyone has experienced the feeling that they are not being listened to, and in this respect it is invariably the non-verbal rather than verbal signs which are the most telling. When verbal and non-verbal messages conflict—for example, if the listener says 'How interesting' while at the same time looking at his or her watch, or opening a magazine— the speaker will believe the non-verbal message. Thus non-verbal communication is of great importance in listening.

3.2.3 Questioning

There are basically two types of questions—open or closed. To illustrate the difference, if a pharmacist was going to advise a patient about how to stop smoking, an open question would be 'Tell me about your smoking', and the equivalent closed questions might be a series such as 'When do you smoke?', 'How many do you smoke a day?', 'Where do you smoke?', 'Why do you want to stop?', and so on.

Open questions are known to produce lengthier answers and can thus be more time-consuming for the pharmacist. However, such questions encourage the expression of feelings, attitudes, and emotions. In the context of health promotion, such questions can produce information which helps the pharmacist to better understand the patient's goals and motives. Typical opening phrases might be 'Can you tell me about . . .?', 'Can you describe . . .'.

One approach which can be taken is the 'funnel' technique where the pharmacist begins with one or two open questions and then gradually narrows the focus of the consultation by asking a series of less open questions. Such an approach has much to commend it in response to symptoms. In reply to a question such as 'What's the best thing for a headache?', a pharmacist using a funnelling technique might first ask 'Can you tell me about the headache?' or 'What's the headache like?', thus inviting the customer to give their views and thoughts. The pharmacist's subsequent line of questioning will be based on information given, summarizing and checking, allowing the focus of questioning to be developed. The focus of later questions will thus narrow—for example, 'So you've been having the headaches for about a week and it hurts all around your head. Have you noticed any other symptoms before or during the headache?', 'Are you taking any medicines?', 'Can you think of anything that might be causing the headaches?'. Then 'So you haven't had any other problems like feeling sick, and you're not taking any other medicines, but you've been very busy at work recently' . . . , and so on.

3.2.4 Explaining skills

Pharmacists often give patients many items of information in an unstructured way during explaining and advice-giving. In fact research in community pharmacies and elsewhere has shown that most people will only remember three or four items of information from a verbal explanation, so it is imperative that a way is found to emphasize the most important facts and also ensure that the list of facts is kept as short as possible. In this context, the supplementation of verbal information by written leaflets can be extremely helpful, and leaflets can be used to point out the most important pieces of information.

Generally, a valuable structure for explanations is as follows:

1. introduction (what and why)

2. information, and

3. summary

In such a sequence, the pharmacist will begin by introducing the explanation which is to be given and then briefly show its relevance and importance. For example, 'I'm going to tell you how to increase the fibre in your diet. This will help to stop your constipation coming back. This leaflet shows you the three easiest ways to increase fibre in the diet . . .'. And then, 'So, just to run through that again, there are three points and they are . . .'. Various means can be used to emphasize different pieces of information. Simply by saying 'This is very important', the pharmacist can flag-up the value of the information he is about to give. The use of numbering sequences can be helpful. For example, in the above exchange the pharmacist identifies that there are three pieces of information which are important, and this can further be emphasized by the use of 'Firstly, Secondly, and Thirdly' before each section. Repetition of the most important points is another means of improving patient recall. Finally, a demonstration—for example of how to use an inhaler—can be a most effective way to help understanding.

The pharmacist should invite feedback at the end of any explanation in order to check that the patient has understood. To follow through the example on dietary fibre, the pharmacist might obtain feedback by asking the patient to relate the information to their own diet and give examples of how they might change it. Research in pharmacies shows that, like doctors, pharmacists rarely check whether the information they have given has been understood and this is undoubtedly an area for improvement.

3.2.5 Influencing/persuading skills

In trying to persuade people to adopt healthy behaviours, the credibility in the eyes of the customer is central to the success of the pharmacist's intervention. We have said that skills in persuading and influencing are essential, and the list below contains factors that can help the development of these skills.

Guidelines for becoming a 'persuasive pharmacist'

1. Consider your personal appearance—do you dress and look like a professional? First impressions are crucial in developing positive expectations among the public.

2. Consider the appearance of your pharmacy—does it have the look and atmosphere of a professional environment? How might you change it?

3. Raise your status and credibility by providing high quality services and information to individuals and to local groups and causes. Take opportunities to show your expertise—for example, by acting as a source of advice to local newspapers and other media.

4. When talking to patients, try to find something in their background that is similar to yours—people are more persuasive if they are perceived as having something in common with their customers.

5. Use simple language and offer as much information as the customer or patient wants.

6. When patients present ideas that do not coincide with yours, give them additional ideas and viewpoints to think about. When a list of opposing views is presented to someone, the last one tends to be the most persuasive and remembered.

7. Strong statements tend to be less effective than a series of milder ones. Involve the patient in formulating an action plan rather than trying to enforce your own plan. A negotiated series of actions is more likely to be followed.

8. When presenting a series of facts or emotional appeals, also present a summary and conclusion, rather than leaving the patient to draw their own conclusions.

9. Remember that, over time, even the most persuasive behaviour and attitude changes tend to diminish. Invite the
customer to return and discuss progress and reinforce changed
behaviours to prolong their effects. Praise effort, progress, and
achievement, however small.

10. Be patient—sometimes the desired change in attitude or behaviour is not readily apparent and it may take some time.

11. State clearly what your intention is—that is, the behaviour
change needed at the beginning of your persuasive argument.

12. Find a positive value, attitude, or behaviour held by the patient
and express positive feelings about it. Develop this positive
aspect and use it in your persuasive approach.

(Adapted from *Communication skills in pharmacy practice*,
Tindall *et al.* 1989

3.2.6 Written information

Undoubtedly, written information can be an effective way to reinforce and supplement verbal explanations. Currently some, but
not all, prescription products contain patient leaflets. The potential
for computerized labelling systems to generate personalized leaflets
is beginning to be exploited. Some pharmacists stock a range of
leaflets specific to certain drug groups (e.g. antibiotics) or dosage
forms (e.g. eye drops or suppositories). All these developments are
to be welcomed, but it is important to recognize that, even when
designed and distributed with the best of intentions, the leaflet may
not be read by the patient, and even if read, may not be understood
or remembered.

Research and experience have shown that the kind of written
information used is crucial to success. The type and complexity of
language used are major factors—the average reading age of the
British population is around six years. One expert suggested that
the language used should resemble that in the most commonly-read
daily tabloids—the *Sun* and the *Daily Mirror*—since that was the
kind of written information many members of the public would be
familiar with. We have already discussed (pp. 47–8) the use of
jargon and terms with which members of the public have been
shown to be unfamiliar.

The typeface used must be sufficiently large to allow it to be read by those with poor or fading eyesight. Layout and the use of illustrations have also been found to influence whether a leaflet is read. There is no point in having leaflets containing excellent information if they will not be read by the intended audience.

One way in which pharmacists can increase the likelihood of the leaflet being read by the patient is to incorporate the contents of the leaflet into the explanation. The length of time taken in the verbal explanation may then be reduced, by pointing out only the most important features. Examples of effective use could be:

I'm going to give you the results of your cholesterol test. Your figure was 5.5 and you can see from the table on this leaflet that it's not too high. But it's still important that you eat a healthy diet, and the main ways to do that are here on this page . . .

Here's a leaflet about the sun and skin cancer. There are three important things to remember and they're shown here. The first is that you must make sure you don't get sunburned, so you need a good lotion or cream to wear in the sun . . .

Here's the leaflet that tells you how to use your new inhaler. I'll show you how to use it and go through the leaflet with you to point out the most important parts. You start by shaking the inhaler like this . . .

The pharmacist should, therefore, carefully select the leaflets stocked and read them for their appropriateness. A knowledge of the content of each leaflet will make it easier to incorporate the leaflet into the explanation given. When the supply of 'Pharmacy Healthcare' scheme leaflets arrives, it's a good idea to spend a few minutes reading the leaflet and thinking how you might use it in explanations. The Health Education Authority or your local Health Promotion Unit can advise on which leaflets are available and can provide stocks. The 'Pharmacy Healthcare' scheme will continue to supply a range of leaflets to pharmacies. As we have said, using leaflets in this way can both help the patient's understanding and recall, and reduce the amount of time spent by the pharmacist in giving the explanation.

3.2.7 Maximizing patients' understanding and memory

To summarize what we have said, there are simple ways in which pharmacists can increase customers' memory and understanding of the health promotion advice they are given. A summary of effective information-giving is given below.

- Speak slowly

- Avoid jargon

- Use short words and sentences—simplification

- Increase recall—minimise the number of facts given
  —select the most important
  —stress importance
  —specific rather than general
  —repetition

- Written back-up—readability
  —physical format—type size, colour, quality, of print and paper
  —Link with verbal information

- Encourage feedback—check understanding

  (adapted from *Communicating with patients*, Ley)

3.3 The pharmacy environment — what changes are needed?

3.3.1 Consultation areas

The creation of a private area for talking to patients is one of the most effective changes which the pharmacist could make. The existence of such an area will help to increase the degree of privacy available and may encourage patients to talk to the pharmacist about subjects which are potentially sensitive or embarrassing. Increasingly, shopfitting companies are developing expertise in making the best use of even small areas of space for this purpose. The inclusion of a 'quiet spot' in new pharmacies or refitted premises is strongly encouraged by the National Pharmaceutical Association. If your pharmacy is to be refitted, consider asking for advice about consultation areas—by using imaginative design and, layout (and, sometimes, screens) success has been achieved in many pharmacies with relatively few structural changes required.

    Where a refit is not feasible, at least in the immediate future, the pharmacist needs to give careful thought to how privacy might be increased. Thus, it is important for pharmacists to consider how such privacy can be created within their pharmacy environment. Some pharmacists have a separate consulting room in their premises, either where a room already existed or where the pharmacy has been redesigned. However, refitting is not always feasible and the financial outlay required may be prohibitive. Some pharmacists feel that a separate room is not the answer to the problem of privacy. They argue that, while in such a room, the pharmacist finds it more difficult to remain aware of other transactions occurring in the shop, and is thus unable to fulfil the requirements of supervision of activities such as the sale of 'Pharmacy Only' medicines. So long as the majority of pharmacies employ only one pharmacist, this will remain a potential problem. It has also been argued that the presence of a consulting room alters the essentially informal atmosphere within the pharmacy and that customers may not wish to use such a room. Recent Royal Pharmaceutical Society guidelines on cholesterol measurement require a room separate from the dispensary for the service to be undertaken. The increasing number of pharmacies planning to undertake this and other screening tests will mean that a greater number of pharmacy premises may have the facility of a separate consulting room in the future.

Where a separate room is not available, the identification of a quiet area labelled 'Consultation Area' or 'Advice from the Pharmacist', sometimes with a dividing screen from the rest of the counter or pharmacy, can be helpful.

Some pharmacists invite the patient into the dispensary when discussing a sensitive or private subject. However, the security implications of doing so must be considered and may sometimes preclude such action. At the most basic level, simply going around the counter to the same side as the patient will remove the barrier which the counter can present. Most pharmacies have a quieter area or corner where conversations can be conducted away from other customers, and this is one option where a designated counselling area or room is not available.

3.3.2 Health promotion literature

We would encourage pharmacists to stock a range of leaflets. Displaying and using those included in the 'Pharmacy Healthcare' scheme is important in continuing the nationally-coordinated provision of information. Pharmacists, by forming and developing links with their local Health Promotion Unit and Health Promotion Officer, can identify and take part in local initiatives and campaigns. Stocking a small range of additional leaflets on, for example, commonly-encountered areas such as smoking and diet, can support and reinforce the advice given by the pharmacist. While recognizing the difficulties in identifying space for effective display of literature, it should be possible in any pharmacy to find room for a leaflet stand. Where space permits, the display of posters on health promotion topics is another means of attracting attention to this aspect of the pharmacist's role and provoking interest and questions from customers. Some pharmacies have a 'health notice board', to draw attention to local initiatives, which can be used by community and self-help groups to publicize activities. Your local Health Promotion Unit should be able to help with supplies of posters and leaflets.

3.3.3 Screening services

For those pharmacists who wish to develop them, screening services will undoubtedly be of interest to customers. Pharmacists need to recognize that, for such tests to be carried out, a separate, private area of the pharmacy will be required, and this can be considered if and when the pharmacy is refitted should current facilities be inadequate. Screening tests can form a focus for health promotion advice but are not to be undertaken lightly. In Chapter 5 of this book we will discuss the ethical, training, quality and practical issues relating to screening.

3.3.4 Pharmacist knowledge and skills

The display of health promotion leaflets and posters, and the provision of screening services, will undoubtedly result in increasing numbers of requests for information and advice from pharmacy customers. It is imperative that pharmacists possess the appropriate knowledge and skills to be able to provide a high quality service.

In this chapter we have discussed the importance of interpersonal skills in offering advice on health matters. We will now go on to underpin this with the knowledge base relating to ill health and its prevention in specific areas.

4 Preventing coronary heart disease

Coronary heart disease is at epidemic levels in the UK. In this chapter we will look at the epidemiology of heart disease, at the major risk factors, and at practical advice which the pharmacist can offer customers who wish to reduce their risk. The individual involved may have several risk factors and pharmacists should be aware that it may be necessary to tackle one of these at a time, prioritizing those which have the greatest potential to positively influence health. Care must be taken not to overload people with too much information and advice at one time. With the increasing provision of blood pressure measurement and cholesterol measuring tests in community pharmacies, the pharmacist has a focus to offer health education advice in the prevention of coronary heart disease.

4.1 Epidemiology

In 1987, 178 000 British men and women died from coronary heart disease, making it the leading cause of death in the UK, responsible for the deaths of one in three men and one in four women. Coronary heart disease is the major cause of premature death; one in every four men who die from it do so before the age of 65. There is significant geographical variation in death rates from coronary heart disease in the UK, with the highest in Northern Ireland, Scotland, and the north of England.

The enormous costs of the epidemic of heart disease are difficult to calculate but, in addition to the personal cost in individual and family suffering, the financial cost to the nation is huge. The Office of Health Economics estimated that, for 1985–6, heart disease cost the NHS close to £400 million. Estimates for 1979 suggest that coronary heart disease led to the loss of 26 million working days in that year alone. In 1989 a government minister stated that treatment of coronary heart disease in the NHS was estimated to cost £500 million per year.

Table 4.1 Death rates per 100 000 from coronary heart disease, 1987 (Men aged 35–74)†

Scotland	655
Northern Ireland	634
Finland	593
Czechoslovakia	560
England and Wales	512
Sweden	418
Australia	391
USA	355
Germany	341
Switzerland	238
Portugal	155
France	148
Japan	62

† Age standardized (35–74) to England and Wales population 1972.
(Source: Coronary Prevention Group/British Heart Foundation Statistics Database 1989)

Currently, Northern Ireland, Scotland, England and Wales have death rates from heart disease which are among the highest in the world (Table 4.1).

Of particular cause for concern is the fact that in the UK, whilst there has been a small fall in the death rate from heart disease in recent years, there has been little progress in substantially reducing morbidity and mortality from this cause. This is in stark contrast to countries such as the USA and Australia, where health promotion programmes during the last two decades have led to significant falls in mortality and created high public awareness of risk factors for heart disease and the necessary lifestyle changes. During the period 1970 to 1980, death rates from coronary heart disease fell by over 30 per cent in the USA and Australia. This fall was substantially higher than for the UK, where the equivalent figure was nearer 10 per cent (Table 4.2).

Heart disease was once viewed as a problem of affluent societies and a disease of the rich. Until the 1950s deaths from coronary heart disease occurred more frequently in the higher social classes. Today, the incidence of heart disease is far higher among the poorest sections of our society than among the richest. While research evidence suggests that social class differences in heart disease are largely attributable to smoking levels within these groups, there are other differences which will be discussed later in this chapter, including exercise and important aspects of nutrition. There are few social class differences in fat intake as a percentage of energy, for example. However, fruit and vegetable consumption is higher in the higher socioeconomic groups.

Heart disease affects all socioeconomic groups but the highest death rates are found in the lower socioeconomic groups, that is among manual workers (Table 4.3). It is noteworthy that a larger percentage in this group smoke than in higher socioeconomic groups, where the health risks from smoking were recognized and acted upon some years ago.

The continuing overall reduction in the percentage of the population who smoke, and thus in cigarette consumption, is thought to have contributed to the decline in death rates from heart disease which is now beginning to emerge. The National Food Survey has tracked the British diet over a period of several decades and clearly shows that the diet has improved in some respects. The amount of wholemeal bread purchased has risen, as has that of skimmed and semi-skimmed milks, with a corresponding reduction in the amount of full-fat milk consumed. More poultry is consumed, with relatively less red meat. However, it should be noted that the National Food Survey does not include foods eaten outside the home, so that snacks and take-away food eaten at work or while out of the home do not appear in the figures.

Concern has been expressed that the UK does not yet have a national screening programme for heart disease, and the recent

Table 4.2 Death rates from coronary heart disease 1970–85 by country

	1970	1975	1980	1985
England and Wales	588	611	587	554
Northern Ireland	748	747	761	689
Scotland	728	741	707	687
Australia	758	654	523	442
USA	757	678	491	401

Rates are per 100 000 for men aged 35–74.
Age standardized to England and Wales population 1972.
(Source: Coronary Prevention Group/British Heart Foundation Statistics Database 1989)

Table 4.3 Deaths from coronary heart disease by social class in Great Britain

Social class	Type of occupation	Deaths per 1000	Standardized mortality ratio
I	Professional	1.2	70
II	Intermediate	1.7	82
IIIN	Skilled non-manual	2.1	104
IIIM	Skilled manual	2.1	109
IV	Partly-skilled manual	2.7	112
V	Unskilled manual	3.5	144

Men aged 20–64, ICD codes 410–4.
(Source: OPCS (1986) *Occupational mortality, Decennial supplement*)

emphasis on health promotion within primary healthcare should help to ensure that accurate recording in medical notes of smoking, diet, exercise, and alcohol consumption is carried out. The National Forum for Coronary Heart Disease Prevention has recommended that the Department of Health should ensure that a national information system is established to monitor major coronary risk factors and related behaviours, as has been done already in the USA and Australia.

4.2 Major risk factors

Coronary heart disease is the result of atherosclerosis, where deposits of cholesterol and other lipids lead to thickening of artery walls. Gradually blood flow is restricted as the lumen of the blood vessel becomes progressively narrower. Many factors influence whether an individual will develop coronary heart disease and the rate at which atherosclerosis progresses.

The most important risk factors for heart disease are cigarette smoking, high blood cholesterol, and high blood pressure, all of which have been shown to have a causal effect. Other risk factors include obesity, diabetes, physical inactivity, and heavy alcohol consumption (see below). Genetic predisposition, increasing age, and gender are recognised factors which cannot be altered by behaviour change. Recent work has provided strengthening of the evidence that psycho-social factors also play an important role.

Some risk factors are amenable to amendment by behaviour

change and the pharmacist needs to know the necessary changes sought.

Risk factors for coronary heart disease

Fixed	*Modifiable*
Gender (being male)	Cigarette smoking
Family history	Raised blood cholesterol
Age (middle-aged and older)	Hypertension
Diabetes	Obesity
	Alcohol consumption
	Physical inactivity
	Stress

4.2.1 Cigarette smoking

This will be discussed in detail in Chapter 7 and is the single most important risk factor for coronary heart disease. One in four of all deaths from coronary heart disease have been estimated to be due to smoking. Stopping smoking is the single most important lifestyle change which an individual can make to reduce the risk of heart disease, and even those who have already had a heart attack can reduce their future risk by stopping smoking. For those smokers who have had a myocardial infarction the risk of death from subsequent infarctions is reduced by half in those who stop compared with those who carry on smoking. Smoking particularly increases the risk of heart disease in younger people—those aged under 45 who smoke 25 or more cigarettes a day are 15 times more likely to die from heart disease as are non-smokers.

When discussing smoking with customers, pharmacists often encounter 'old chestnuts' such as the argument that relatives and friends smoked heavily for years without adverse effects. Statistically, the facts show clearly that for the majority smoking is extremely harmful to health. Pharmacy customers, and particularly women, may say that stopping smoking will lead to an increase in weight. This should be countered by a strong statement that cigarette smoking is infinitely more dangerous to health than is being overweight. In any case, after an initial weight gain in some individuals, there appears to be no long-term evidence that stopping smoking will in itself increase weight. The pharmacist can offer healthy eating advice to offset any potential weight gain.

4.2.2 Cholesterol

The level of cholesterol in the blood is strongly related to an individual's risk of coronary heart disease. Research has shown that the 20 per cent of people who have the highest cholesterol levels are three times more likely to die from heart disease than the 20 per cent with the lowest levels. It has been estimated that a 10 per cent reduction in blood cholesterol is associated with a 20–30 per cent reduction in heart disease.

When trying to define the population at risk, attempts have been made to identify the cholesterol level below which there is no risk of heart disease. The World Health Organization concluded that a cholesterol level of 5.2 mmol/litre or less is associated with a lower risk of heart disease in people aged over 30, and for people under 30 the appropriate equivalent level is 4.7 mmol/litre. Studies have shown that, based on those guidelines, over half the British population is at risk of heart disease. Any strategy for reducing cholesterol levels must, therefore, be aimed at the public in general rather than only those at highest risk.

Blood cholesterol levels are closely related to intake of saturated fats. Originally it was thought that foods which are high in cholesterol were the cause of the problem, but we now understand more clearly that a diet which is high in saturated fat leads to high blood cholesterol levels and the associated risk. HDL (high-density lipoprotein) cholesterol appears to have a protective effect against heart disease and a reduced HDL level is associated with a higher risk. A high LDL (low-density lipoprotein) cholesterol relative to HDL, on the other hand, is associated with increased risk. The levels of HDL and LDL are to some extent determined by genetic makeup, although eating patterns are also very important.

In offering advice about blood cholesterol the pharmacist should remember that currently the percentage of total calorie intake which comes from fat is around 42 per cent. Recommendations relating to fat intake differ slightly between the Committee on Medical Aspects of Food (COMA) and World Health Organization. They are listed below:

- No more than 35 per cent (COMA)/30 per cent (WHO) of total calorie intake from fats

- Less than 15 per cent (COMA)/10 per cent (WHO) of total calories from saturated fats

- Dietary intake coupled with exercise sufficient to reach and maintain a desirable body weight

Publicity about the claimed effectiveness of oatbran in reducing blood cholesterol levels was followed by scrutiny of research findings. The lipid-lowering effects of oatbran and other fibrous foods is due, at least in part, to their being included in diets in place of fatty foods. The soluble fibre in pulses, oats, fruit, and vegetables may lead to some reduction in cholesterol, but dietary advice should emphasize reduction in fat levels, particularly saturated fat. This lowered fat intake should be replaced by fibre-rich starchy foods.

The pharmacist can provide leaflets on cholesterol levels and on ways of reducing the amount of fat in the diet. This is discussed in greater detail in Chapter 9 on nutrition (see p. 135) and also summarized in Appendix 1 (see p. 197).

Cholesterol measurement in pharmacies

The availability of high street cholesterol testing to members of the public has been a controversial topic. A King's Fund Consensus statement in 1989 opposed mass screening on the basis that cholesterol measurement taken in isolation did not address the wider range of risk factors for heart disease and the necessary lifestyle changes to reduce risk. However, consumers apparently wanted such a service, and their growing awareness of blood cholesterol and its association with heart disease created a need for on-demand cholesterol tests. A more recent Standing Medical Advisory Committee (SMAC) report supported opportunistic cholesterol testing.

In the USA cholesterol testing is available in shopping malls and retail outlets and is often carried out by personnel with no background in healthcare. During 1989 cholesterol testing became more widely available in the UK, through a small number of pharmacies, in a pilot scheme organized by the Pharmaceutical Services Negotiating Committee (PSNC), and concurrently through branches of the 'health food' multiple, Holland and Barrett. The Holland and Barrett scheme was the subject of criticism from pharmacists and others because of its commercial association with sales of oatbran and niacin (claimed to reduce cholesterol levels) to clients.

Pharmacists who took part in the PSNC trial undertook special training in carrying out the tests, quality assurance measures, heart disease risk factors, and associated advice-giving. Those members of the public who requested a test were asked about other coronary heart disease risk factors and counselled appropriately. Referral to the general practitioner was made on the basis of a strict protocol based on European Atherosclerosis Society guidelines. The scheme was popular with the public, with an average of 26 people per pharmacy each week requesting tests during the study period. The results showed that 61 per cent of the 2171 people tested had a level of greater than 5.2 mmol/litre and 21 per cent greater than 6.5 mmol/litre (the level at which referral to the general practitioner was initiated). Levels between 5.2 and 6.5 mmol/litre were found in 40 per cent of clients, and here advice on dietary measures was given, together with information on other risk factors where present, and the person was invited to return after several months for a second test and to monitor progress. The measurement of cholesterol provided a focus for general health education advice about reducing the risk of heart disease. For pharmacists who are considering setting up a cholesterol measuring service, the ethical, training and other issues are discussed in the next chapter. The argument about high street testing continues, but many pharmacists consider that if such testing is to be done (and the consumer demand is apparent) then it is better done in a healthcare environment such as a pharmacy, where the pharmacist has wide knowledge about the issues involved and can offer advice in a professional setting.

Lipid-lowering drugs versus dietary measures

There is debate about the role of drug treatments and diet in the reduction of cholesterol levels. Experts are agreed that the desired change is in lifestyle and that the treatment of raised blood cholesterol levels should always begin with dietary advice. Only where dietary changes made over a period of several months have not produced the required fall in blood cholesterol should drug treatment be commenced. Many health educators hold the view that drug treatment should be reserved for those with familial hypercholesterolaemia and those in whom prolonged dietary measures have been insufficient. The concern is that drug treatment will be seen as an easier option than modifying diet and lifestyle, and the pharmacist has an important role as a health educator in advising customers to make changes towards healthier eating. Quite apart from the principle that lifestyle change is the more healthy approach, drug treatment is very expensive and the long-term effects, particularly of the newer classes of lipid-lowering drugs, are not yet known.

A 1989 Royal Society of Medicine meeting on dietary fat and heart disease concluded that barriers to progress included a fatalistic attitude on the part of the public, particularly amongst those at risk and the less well-off. This is illustrated by research which showed that, whilst over two-thirds of professional and managerial classes felt that they could reduce their chances of having a heart attack, less than half of those in the manual and unskilled worker group agreed with this statement. The difficulties of attempting to persuade people of the benefit of making dietary changes when the benefits would not be seen for perhaps another 30 years were also cited. The meeting identified that most medical schools have no department of nutrition and that the subject is under-taught in medical courses. The same comments apply currently to many schools of pharmacy. Finally, in addition to a lack of coordination among the major organizations involved with coronary heart disease, and a lack of monitoring of risk factors, the meeting identified the problem of mixed messages being provided to members of the public, which frequently seem to be in conflict. Thus, those research reports or scientists' views which are against the current thinking that diet is important in coronary heart disease often receive wide publicity in the popular press.

4.2.3 Hypertension

Hypertension is a major risk factor in coronary heart disease and is a largely asymptomatic condition, hence it is often only discovered through opportunistic or structured screening programmes. Raised blood pressure is known to be associated with both coronary heart disease and stroke. The so-called 'Rule of Halves' applies to hypertension, which says that:

- only half of those with hypertension are identified;
- only half of these are treated;
- hypertension is controlled in only half those who are treated.

Recent large-scale population studies in the UK have confirmed the 'Rule of Halves' to be correct.

There is debate about the level at which anti-hypertensive treatment should be initiated, since studies have shown that the treatment of mild hypertension reduces the number of deaths from stroke but not coronary heart disease. The case for the treatment of hypertension to prevent coronary heart disease is certainly not so strong as is the case for stopping smoking. Any reduction in heart disease achieved by reducing blood pressure would potentially be substantial because of the large number of people with raised blood pressure. While blood pressure rises with increasing age in the developed countries, this is not the case in developing countries, and there is an urgent need to try to prevent the rise in blood pressure which then contributes to coronary risk. This might be achieved by lifestyle changes such as dietary change, weight reduction, stopping smoking, and reducing stress, and these approaches might initially be tried before medication is introduced. Sodium restriction can help to reduce blood pressure in some hypertensives. Long-term anti-hypertensive medication can itself produce effects which contribute to the development of heart disease, such as adverse changes in blood lipids.

Blood pressure measurement in the pharmacy

A small percentage of pharmacies (5 per cent in one large city studied in 1985) offer a blood pressure measurement service. Such a service gives the pharmacist the opportunity to offer screening for high blood pressure and also to monitor the effectiveness of and compliance with anti-hypertensive treatment. Several studies have been conducted in community pharmacies which have shown the service to be feasible and welcomed by the public. The professional satisfaction to be derived from identifying those who are hypertensive, and later monitoring progress, was found to be high among those pharmacists who took part.

The Royal Pharmaceutical Society has produced guidelines for those pharmacists who wish to provide a blood pressure measuring service (see Chapter 5, p. 86). Of particular importance are the recommended levels above which the client should be referred to his or her general practitioner for further investigation. Communication with local medical practices is important when any screening or diagnostic testing service is to be offered through the pharmacy. We suggest that pharmacists should inform local doctors of the service they intend to provide and agree the protocol and levels for referral.

Lifestyle changes—such as stopping smoking, reducing alcohol intake, and eating more healthily—can contribute towards a reduction in blood pressure. With advice from the pharmacist, these can be tried before other interventions, such as drug therapy, are made. Offering written information in conjunction with verbal advice is valuable. As with any health education advice, an invitation to the person to return to monitor progress is important.

4.2.4 Obesity

Middle-aged people who are in the heaviest 20 per cent of the population have double the coronary risk of those in the lowest 20 per cent. Body Mass Index (BMI) is a more useful indicator of obesity than is weight alone. BMI is calculated as weight (kg)/height (m) squared. The resulting figure can be classified as shown below:

Body Mass Index and obesity

	BMI
	BMI
'Underweight'	20 or less
'Average'	over 20 to 25
'Overweight'	over 25 to 30
'Obese'	over 30

Obesity has been increasing in the UK over the last 50 years and the 1990 Dietary and Nutritional Survey of British Adults showed 45 per cent of males and 36 per cent of females to be overweight, with one in twelve men and one in eight women classified as obese. These figures showed a significant increase in the percentages of the population classified as overweight and obese since the last survey, reported in 1980. Since those who are overweight often consume a diet which is high in fats, lipid levels are correspondingly high. Blood pressure is also raised in those who are overweight. Those who are overweight tend to take less exercise. All these factors increase the risk of coronary heart disease.

In addition to the raised lipid levels mentioned earlier, people who are fat have a greater risk of coronary heart disease because their increased weight puts a greater strain on the heart. Being overweight is also associated with an increase in blood pressure and in serum cholesterol and a decrease in physical activity. The benefits of reducing weight are that the work-load of the heart is reduced, that carbohydrate metabolism is improved (thus lessening the risk of diabetes), and that serum lipid concentrations fall. The message for those who are overweight is to reduce their calorie intake, particularly by reducing saturated fats and sugar, and to increase physical activity. Alcohol intake can provide a significant calorie intake and should be considered and reduced where necessary.

The pharmacist has an important role to play in giving advice about weight reduction to achieve a desirable body weight. Such advice can be strengthened if there is a set of weighing scales in the pharmacy. This means that an accurate and consistent measure of weight is possible and that the person can return to the pharmacy to be re-weighed. In previous years such weighing scales were common in community pharmacies but are now rarely seen. Advice and products for weight reduction are discussed fully in Chapter 9 on nutrition (see p. 140).

4.2.5 Exercise

Current thinking is that, for a protective cardiovascular effect, exercise which increases the heart rate should be taken 3 times a week for around 20 minutes each period. Concern is currently being expressed at the low percentage of people in the UK who undertake any form of regular exercise (Table 4.4), and particularly amongst schoolchildren, where it is thought that the lack of regular physical activity is likely to continue after leaving school, building-up a higher risk of heart disease for the future. One study in Wales in 1985 showed that only one in four adult men undertook very active exercise in work- or leisure-time, and even fewer women (2 per

Table 4.4   Sports, games, and physical activity in men and women aged 16 and over in Great Britain, 1977–86

	1977		1980		1983		1986	
	Men	Women	Men	Women	Men	Women	Men	Women
Outdoor								
At least one activity, excluding walking	23%	8%	24%	9%	26%	10%	27%	10%
At least one activity, including walking	35%	21%	37%	24%	39%	24%	40%	24%
Indoor	31%	13%	32%	15%	33%	18%	35%	21%

(Source: General Household Survey, 1986/Coronary Prevention Group/British Heart Foundation Statistics Database 1989)

cent). Even in the most active group—teenage males—less than half took regular active exercise.

The increase in interest in exercise which has occurred during the last decade is illustrated by the high popularity and demand for sports facilities and use of health clubs. Recent research, though, suggests that the awareness of the need for exercise is highest in the higher socioeconomic groups, who have accepted the message that regular exercise is needed and can help prevent heart disease. Among those in lower socioeconomic groups, the percentage of people who take regular exercise is substantially lower. The highest participation rates in exercise in leisure-time are found among professional and managerial people and their spouses, and the lowest rates are found amongst unskilled workers. Manual workers, however, may undertake very active jobs and thus achieve a high level of activity at work, so this must be taken into account. For the future, with increasing levels of mechanization and reduction in production-based industries in favour of service industries, this effect will be greatly reduced. The National Forum for Coronary Heart Disease Prevention considers that, in the future, leisure-time will provide the major opportunity for exercise promotion for all social groups.

The pharmacist is in a good position to offer advice on taking exercise as part of an overall plan for a healthier lifestyle and is able to explain that exercise—such as brisk walking and swimming—provides cardiovascular benefit, so that the perception that exercise must be vigorous to give any such benefit is mistaken. Current thinking is that the individual should choose the form of exercise which suits them and which they enjoy, so that a long-term change in behaviour is more likely to result. The pharmacist can also emphasize to parents the message that the establishment of regular exercise during childhood and the teenage years can help to make exercise feature as a normal part of everyday life, and again set a pattern for later years. In addition to its cardioprotective effect for women, regular exercise begun at an early age will help to prevent the development of osteoporosis in later life.

4.2.6 Stress

Stress has been much publicized in the media as an important contributory factor to heart disease. Research on personality characteristics produced a classification of Type A and Type B personalities, where the Type A personality was someone who was ambitious, worried a lot, and was thus subject to high levels of stress. People of Type A personality appear to be at higher risk of developing heart disease.

While it has been shown that a reduction in stress levels can help to reduce high blood pressure, in the public's mind the importance of stress as a risk factor is vastly overestimated. Another common public misperception about stress is that its levels are highest in executives—the classic businessman rushing from meeting to meeting. In reality, stress levels are high throughout the range of socioeconomic groups, and research has shown that stress levels in an unskilled worker doing a boring, repetitive job are as high as, or higher than, in professional and managerial groups.

The pharmacist has an important part to play in explaining that the major avoidable risk factors are smoking, high blood pressure, and high blood cholesterol levels. That is not to say that information and advice about stress reduction is not of value. Indeed, some pharmacies stock video and audio cassette tapes which teach relaxation techniques. There may also be local groups and courses aimed at reducing stress.

4.3 Major initiatives in health promotion and the prevention of coronary heart disease

In recent years, Wales has begun its 'Heartbeat Wales' programme, aimed at reducing morbidity and mortality from coronary heart disease. England followed with its 'Look After Your Heart' campaign, and Northern Ireland has its own campaign. All these programmes aim to raise public awareness of the modifiable risk factors for heart disease and to suggest the necessary lifestyle changes. Scotland is currently the only country within the UK that does not have a national programme which is specifically aimed at coronary heart disease, although there have been local initiatives such as the 'Good-Hearted Glasgow' programme.

Heart disease prevention is one of the priority targets of the Health Education Authority, and the new contract for General Medical Practitioners in England requires them to increase the level of screening and health promotion advice which they offer. The community pharmacist has an important role to play in several areas. Firstly, the stocking and display of leaflets about the prevention of heart disease can encourage interest among pharmacy customers and perhaps prompt the asking of questions of the pharmacist. Secondly, the availability of leaflets on specific risk factors—such as smoking, diet, and exercise—can help the pharmacist to base advice for lifestyle change. Thirdly, the provision of testing services—such as cholesterol measurement and blood pressure measurement—and, more simply, the availability of weighing machines and charts for customers to tell whether they are within the ideal weight range for their height, can provide the basis for a great deal of health promotion advice. While measuring cholesterol as a risk factor in isolation from other risk factors has little value, the results of the test can provide a tangible basis for suggesting behaviour change. Cholesterol testing and the advice which follows must always, however, be linked with questioning and advice about the other risk factors for coronary heart disease. For blood pressure measurement, a slightly raised level can provide the basis for advice about dietary modification, weight loss, reduction in alcohol consumption, and smoking cessation. Again, it is important that the pharmacist takes a history which includes other risk factors for heart disease.

PREVENTING CORONARY HEART DISEASE—KEY POINTS

- Stopping cigarette smoking
- Improving eating patterns
- Reducing and maintaining body weight at the ideal weight-for-height ratio
- Promoting regular exercise

In this chapter we have examined the major risk factors for coronary heart disease and the ways in which lifestyle modification can reduce an individual's risk. In the chapters which follow, on smoking and nutrition, more specific guidelines will be given about the kind of practical advice and support which the pharmacist might offer.

5   Screening and diagnostic testing

With the development of desk-top testing equipment, the feasibility of screening and diagnostic testing based in community pharmacies is increasing. Pregnancy testing has been carried out in pharmacies for many years. More recent developments include blood pressure measurement, cholesterol measurement, and the use of peak-flow meters to screen for obstructive airways disease. Whilst the pharmacist's healthcare training provides an appropriate foundation upon which to conduct screening and to advise clients, pharmacists must be specially trained to undertake this developing aspect of their role. In addition, there are important ethical considerations in screening and diagnostic testing which mean that these procedures cannot be undertaken lightly. The pharmacist must always work to a carefully defined protocol and must ensure, by quality assurance procedures, that the screening or testing service being provided is of a high standard.

Screening and testing services which might be provided in community pharmacies

- Pregnancy testing†

- Ovulation testing

- Cholesterol and triglyceride measurement†

- Blood pressure measurement†

- Peak flow testing

- Blood/urine glucose testing

- Body weight/height measurement

†Denotes that Royal Pharmaceutical Society guidelines are available.

5.1 Ethical aspects of screening and diagnostic testing

It is important for the pharmacist to recognize that he or she is a health professional offering a screening service to 'healthy' clients rather than as a response to illness. Apparently healthy clients may request a screening test, the results of which will show that referral for medical advice, and perhaps treatment, is needed. The pharmacist, like any other health professional offering a screening service, has responsibilities in relation to that service. If any abnormality or result outside the normal range exists, then it must be found in the screening procedure—that is to say that the pharmacist must ensure that any equipment used is capable of giving an accurate result, is not likely to give false positives or false negatives, and is constantly maintained and calibrated using reference standards. A false positive says that an abnormality is present when it is not; a false negative means that an abnormality is there but is not identified. A false positive test may cause distress and anxiety, while a false negative result will lead to reassurance and lack of treatment for a condition which may progress.

Criteria have been defined for the adoption of screening for a particular condition. These are shown below.

Criteria for adoption of screening for any condition

- The condition screened for should be an important one

- There should be an acceptable treatment for the disease

- Facilities for diagnosis or treatment should be available

- The disease should have a recognized latent or early symptomatic stage

- A suitable test or examination must exist

- The test or examination should be acceptable to the population

- The natural history of the condition, including its development from a latent to an actual disease, should be adequately understood

- The cost of screening, including diagnosis and subsequent treatment, should be economically balanced in relation to potential benefits

- The screening should be continuous and not a 'one-off' project

(Adapted from *Practising prevention*, Fowler, G.)

Screening for the risk factors of coronary heart disease fulfil most of these criteria. For the future, pharmacists may screen blood or urine for diabetes, which would also meet the criteria. Testing for HIV, while not undertaken in pharmacies, nor likely to be so, does not fulfil several of the main criteria, since no effective treatment is yet available and thus the patient has no hope of the condition being controlled or cured.

Before any test procedure, the pharmacist must give a clear explanation of the benefits to the client and obtain the consent of the client to a test. The test procedure itself should be fully explained so that, for a cholesterol test, the client knows that the taking of a blood sample is involved. The consequences of intervention must also be outlined—that is, if the result falls outside normal limits, it must be made clear that referral by the pharmacist to medical or other expert help will be strongly advised where necessary. In some cases the pharmacist may think it appropriate, with the patient's agreement, to contact the general practitioner while the patient is in the pharmacy. The client's consent must be sought and given before any information is given to the doctor. Confidentiality of information is fundamental to the screening or testing service, and the pharmacist must ensure that the results of any such tests are stored in such a way that they are not accessible either to unauthorized members of staff or to the public.

Pharmacists sometimes express concern about the ethical aspects of charging a fee for a screening test. The Royal Pharmaceutical Society's guidelines on cholesterol and blood pressure measurement indicate clearly that it is *not* unethical to make such a charge.

In any test procedure the pharmacist must ensure that his knowledge is sufficient to carry out the test, interpret the findings, and advise the client accordingly. The pharmacist must know the nature of the health risk involved, normal parameters for the population, referral points and sources of further advice, and details of any lifestyle change required. In addition, the pharmacist must know not only how to use the equipment correctly but also the requirements for servicing and monitoring. The test should be carried out according to recognized guidelines and standards, using a clearly-defined protocol.

The pharmacist's code of ethics requires that the pharmacist should not take any action which would impair the patient's confidence in the prescriber, and a good relationship between the pharmacist, the patient, and their general practitioner must be maintained. It is appropriate, therefore, to inform local GPs about any new service to be offered through the pharmacy and to agree referral points. For example, in the case of measuring blood pressure, agreement should be reached about the systolic and diastolic pressures at which the pharmacist should refer the client to their doctor. That is not to suggest that the pharmacist should request permission from local prescribers to carry out a service but, rather, that they should be kept properly informed. Experience has shown that, if the pharmacy service is carried out to a high standard and referrals are appropriate without raising patient anxiety, any initial concerns expressed by local doctors are rapidly assuaged.

5.2 Screening and testing protocols

The Royal Pharmaceutical Society has produced guidelines on pregnancy testing, blood pressure measurement, and cholesterol measurement which clearly define a recommended procedure (see pp. 86–95). Whatever test is to be performed, the pharmacist should have a written protocol which should take into account the following points:

1. Whether the screening is *open* or *closed*—for example, are people from certain age ranges excluded?; are people on existing treatment to be included or excluded?

2. Agreement reached with local prescribers about referral points for consequent action—for example, the blood pressure levels at which prescribers begin to treat with hypertensives may vary.

3. Privacy is an essential feature of any screening process, and the Royal Pharmaceutical Society's guidelines suggest, for example, that, with the client's agreement, cholesterol testing must be carried out in a room separate from the main shop area and the dispensary. This will ensure that only the pharmacist

and the client will see the result and that the patient is enabled to ask any questions or express their concerns without being overheard by other members of pharmacy staff or by other customers. Ideally this room should be equipped with a sink with hot and cold running water, and sufficient working bench space. Where the procedure is carried out in a separate room, pharmacists might wish to be ultra-cautious and ensure either that the room is in sight of the dispensary or that another member of staff acts as a chaperone. While this may seem extreme, where a test such as blood pressure measurement may occasionally require the removal of some clothing, the presence of an observer may be sensible.

4. The pharmacist must decide whether the test will be offered on a 'walk-in' basis or by prior appointment. To some extent, this may be determined by demand—for example, in the Pharmaceutical Services Negotiating Committee's (PSNC) pilot study for cholesterol measurement it was originally intended that tests would be offered on a 'walk-in' basis, but the level of demand was such that all the pharmacies involved had to establish an appointment system. (Interestingly, the majority of clients kept their appointments).

5. A check-list of any questions to be asked by the pharmacist and all information which is to be obtained from the patient.

6. The timing which is necessary for the test—for example, a rest period before measuring blood pressure.

7. A definition of the pharmacist's explanation of the test, its findings and its benefits, so that each client can be given consistent information.

8. Whether repeat readings are necessary and, if so, under what conditions and time-scale.

9. An invitation to return to discuss the outcomes of advice given by the pharmacist.

10. An outline of the advice or counselling which is to be given by the pharmacist if the test is outside defined limits, including any intervention and advice on lifestyle and behaviour modification.

11. The advice and counselling to be given if the test falls within
    normal limits. For example, in cholesterol measurement, there
    may still be other aspects of lifestyle change that may be
    necessary. That is to say, if a patient smoked 50 cigarettes a day
    but had a low or normal cholesterol level, the pharmacist
    should still counsel the patient about ways of stopping smoking.

The equipment and test materials must be of good quality and
capable of accurate results. Advice on the selection and costs of
appropriate equipment is available from the National Pharmaceutical Association and from regional hospital quality control
laboratory services.

A written record of the test results should be kept—ideally, the
pharmacist should keep one copy, the patient given the second, and
a third available for the GP but only with the patient's permission.
Confidentiality has already been discussed earlier in this chapter,
and the ethical aspects of confidentiality cannot be stressed too
strongly. The pharmacist should not reveal the results of any test to
a patient's GP unless that patient's agreement has been given. For
example, if the pharmacist has carried out a pregnancy test with a
positive result but the patient is unwilling to go and see her doctor,
the pharmacist's code of ethics means that the result cannot be
communicated to the doctor without the patient's consent.

It is important to establish the age of clients presenting for
pregnancy testing and, if the woman is or appears to be under 16,
strenuous efforts should be made to encourage her to discuss a
positive pregnancy test with either her GP or her parents. Rarely, if
it is suspected that news of a positive result may lead to danger to the
life of either mother or fetus, the pharmacist may judge it necessary
to pass on the test result to the appropriate person without the
consent of the client. However, this would only be in exceptional
cases.

5.3 Record-keeping and documentation

The pharmacist is strongly advised to keep a written record of every
test which is performed and we suggest this should be in triplicate
with copies for pharmacy, patient, and GP. An alternative is to have
a duplicate and to use a referral form, with the client's agreement,
to send the information to the GP (the National Pharmaceutical

Association can supply these). The written record should include the name and address of the patient, the date of the test and the test result as the minimum amount of information. The keeping of records is valuable from a legal viewpoint and can substantiate the test result and advice given by the pharmacist.

Pharmacists involved in practice research can use records as the basis for further research: with the agreement of local GPs, and with the patient's agreement to inform the GP of test findings, they may also follow-up patients to ascertain the outcome—for example, whether the patient visited the doctor and, if so, what treatment, if any, was initiated.

Records of screening tests can also be used for professional audit purposes in analysing numbers of tests performed, the range of results, and the advice given. The Royal Pharmaceutical Society's Law Department suggests that test records should be kept for a minimum of three years.

If pharmacists wish to store the results of tests on computer, then the Data Protection Act applies, and if a client so requests at a later date they are entitled to have a copy of their computer record. Care should be taken that unauthorized persons cannot access these records. If records are eventually destroyed this must be done in such a way that confidentiality is preserved—for example, paper records should be shredded.

5.4 Quality assurance of the testing service

The pharmacist must validate the whole testing process. As far as the equipment is concerned, the manufacturers of cholesterol testing equipment, for example, each have their own quality control system, involving a standard calibration of the machine with test samples. Where possible, the pharmacist should subscribe to an external quality assurance scheme—for example, that run by the Wolfson Laboratories in Birmingham for cholesterol testing. The district or regional quality control hospital service can also be a valuable source of information and advice for pharmacists about the choice of testing equipment and about the availability of facilities for quality assurance. The local school of pharmacy will also be able to offer information and advice. Both internal and external quality control measures must be sought. Equipment such as blood pressure measuring machines must be serviced regularly so as to ensure accuracy.

As part of the quality assurance of their service, pharmacists should carry out a regular audit, surveying the test records to ensure adherence to the protocol, to check referral rates, to check the return rate for re-tests and to check the content and quality of the advice given to clients.

5.5 Legal aspects

Pharmacists should check that their professional indemnity insurance arrangements cover the provision of screening tests. The provision of such tests is considered by most companies (including the National Pharmaceutical Association's CDA cover) to fall within the normal range of professional activities of the pharmacist—that is, they are covered by the policy.

Any pharmacist undertaking screening tests will be under 'a duty of care' to the client not to conduct them negligently. This means that it is important to adhere to recognized guidelines such as those published by the Royal Pharmaceutical Society in the provision of any screening or testing service. Such guidelines, together with widely-published reports and manufacturers' literature and instructions, will be taken by the courts as the benchmark for the standard of competence and knowledge of the 'reasonably competent practitioner'. Any pharmacist offering a specialist service must be 'reasonably competent' so to do and may be liable for damages if the service is carried out negligently. This liability applies regardless of whether the pharmacist is newly-registered or approaching retirement. While no such case has yet been brought, the consequences of not detecting a high reading should be considered by the pharmacist. Consent to the procedures involved is also necessary to avoid any possibility of court action for assault (technically battery).

5.6 Patient fears

For many patients a test procedure which may seem routine to a health professional can be a daunting prospect; even though they have requested the screening process, there may still be fears about process and the outcome. Pharmacists should recognize these fears and should never omit the initial counselling about the test and its benefits, to mitigate any worries that the patient may have. Research has shown that screening generates anxiety and concern in some patients even when results are normal, and thus the psychological consequences of screening are significant. It is of critical importance that the results are communicated in an unemotional and unambiguous way and that, should referral be required, the pharmacist makes this clear to the patient in a way which is not alarming. The importance of privacy in communicating test results has been discussed in Chapter 3 with other important issues in communication.

5.7 Training and updating

The pharmacist must receive training in the use of the appropriate equipment and its quality control. The pharmacist must decide whether anyone else is to perform the tests and, if so, those people should undergo the training process. The health risks which lead to the screening test should be studied—for example, pharmacists should understand the risk factors for coronary heart disease, their relative importance, and the changes which can be made to modify and reduce risk.

The pharmacist must be clear about the behaviour change sought. That is to say, if dietary advice is to be given, the outcomes of such advice must be clear—for example, a reduction in serum cholesterol, a reduction in blood pressure. Counselling skills are of vital importance in any screening or testing procedure, and pharmacists' training should incorporate these skills, preferably by the use of guided role-play. Having undergone intitial training, pharmacists must ensure that the service being provided is the most up-to-date possible by regular reading of journals and equipment manufacturers' manuals so that they can be confident that the advice which they are giving, the referral levels which are being used, and the maintenance and calibration of equipment, are all to an acceptable professional standard. Again, the 'duty of care' concept applies to the standard of knowledge and skills possessed by the pharmacist. In many areas of health promotion expert consensus can change within a matter of months, and it is essential that the pharmacist is abreast with the latest thinking about referral levels, the initiation of drug treatment, and the role of, for example, dietary advice.

5.8 Economic aspects

In setting up any testing service, the pharmacist must consider the financial and economic aspects, including the cost of the equipment, the costs of testing and, in particular, the cost of the pharmacist's time in performing the test and counselling the patient. The cost of quality control measures must also be taken into account. The fee which is charged for the service is to be decided by the pharmacist and will probably be influenced by national averages.

A common problem in health promotion is that it seldom reaches those at highest risk, and pharmacists should therefore be aware of the socioeconomic status and profile of the clients they are screening in order to establish whether their service is meeting the needs of the target groups and those people who need it. Anecdotal evidence from the PSNC's cholesterol pilot study suggests that some less well-off pharmacy customers were reluctant or unable to pay the fee of £6.00 which was being charged at that time. These factors must be balanced with the economic aspects of the service in deciding the fee to be charged. In all probability these will vary slightly from one area to another, but so long as the service is run as a private initiative—that is, without any financial support or input from the Department of Health—patients will continue to bear the entire cost of the test.

5.9 Royal Pharmaceutical Society guidelines

5.9.1 Blood pressure measurement in the pharmacy (Published in the *Pharmaceutical Journal*, July 1986)

The following guidelines have been drawn up by the Royal Pharmaceutical Society for use by pharmacists in connection with apparatus used in pharmacies for the measurement of blood pressure. They have been drawn up on the assumption that the Department of Health will take no immediate action on the Society's recommendation to the Department that such apparatus should be controlled. The Society has recommended that control should be achieved by licensing the apparatus, controlling its siting, and requiring its use to be supervised by suitably qualified persons.

Two sets of guidelines have been prepared: one covers the unassisted use of an automatic apparatus for the measurement of blood pressure by a patient; the second set covers the use of an apparatus by which the pharmacist himself makes the measurement of blood pressure. In the latter circumstances, the pharmacist has direct contact with the patient in every case.

The case for making apparatus for the measurement of blood pressure widely available is that, by screening with such apparatus, cases of mild, symptomless hypertension can be detected. There has been growing support for the medical view, based mainly on considerable experience in the United States, that, if mild hypertension is detected and the patient advised to make appropriate changes in his living habits, for example to reduce his weight and cut down on smoking, or is given long-term treatment with suitable anti-hypertensive drugs, then further increase in blood pressure, which could ultimately lead to death by stroke, congestive heart failure, and probably renal failure, can be averted. If that view be accepted, it has seemed logical to the Council that the pharmacy is a suitable place for the screening to take place. Automatic apparatus by which a patient can measure his own blood pressure could be used, although some pharmacists may wish to be involved in the measurement of blood pressure themselves, using one of the semi-automatic electronic sphygmomanometers which have come on to the market in recent years.

The Council has accepted from the beginning of its discussion on the subject that a screening service could be conducted with the support and advice of the medical profession at national and local level. Such collaboration has been obtained at local level by a few pharmacists who already offer a service, but so far the British Medical Association has not responded to the Society's suggestions for collaboration at national level. In fact, the association has opposed a pilot scheme in which local doctors and pharmacists were prepared to collaborate.

At the time of drawing up these guidelines there is available automatic apparatus by which a patient can measure his own blood pressure. Some apparatus is available on leasing terms. At least one type is operated by a 50p coin; clear directions for use are given on this apparatus; information on blood pressure, interpretation of readings, and when to consult a doctor are given in the manufacturer's leaflet; and a card is supplied on which the blood pressure readings can be recorded. Although it is undesirable there is no reason why, in the absence of any restrictive action by the Department of Health, such apparatus should not be widely distributed in places such as airport lounges, sports centres, and a variety of retail premises. Members of the Society may, in these circumstances, consider that it is irrational and places an unnecessary burden on them to be expected to follow any guidelines when elsewhere there is no supervision whatsoever. However, the Council feels that pharmacists who install such apparatus must act in a responsible and professional way. By doing so, it is hoped that possible difficulties which could arise between doctors and pharmacists over blood pressure measurements can be minimized.

Guidelines for the measurement of blood pressure by a pharmacist with a manually-operated electronic sphygmomanometer

1. The apparatus It is important that the apparatus should be accurate, robust, simple to operate, and easy to clean and maintain under the conditions of use in the pharmacy. The readings of blood pressure should be clearly displayed. Manufacturers of the apparatus should be asked to produce evidence from trials that high readings of blood pressure obtained from the apparatus have subsequently been confirmed by readings taken in doctors' surgeries. If a patient requires his blood pressure to be checked regularly during a course of treatment, it may be best to suggest to him that the readings are taken by the same pharmacist on the same apparatus, thereby eliminating apparatus and operator variations. The pharmacist should ensure that the suppliers of the apparatus provide a regular service to maintain the apparatus and to check its performance.

2. Advertising the apparatus A discreet notice relating to blood pressure screening may be displayed at any pharmacy.

3. Where the apparatus is used It is recommended that the measurement of blood pressure should be carried out in a separate room or cubicle so that the measurement and any discussion of the reading can take place in confidence.

4. *Use of the apparatus* The apparatus should be used in accordance with the manufacturer's instructions. The reading of blood pressure should be recorded on a card or form. As there is an increase of the normal diastolic blood pressure with age, the pharmacist should ascertain the patient's age group and only refer the patient to his doctor if the diastolic blood pressure exceeds the figure for the particular age group given in the following table.

Age (years)	Diastolic blood pressure reading (mm Hg)
30–40	90
40–50	95
50–60	100
60–70	105
Over 70	110

5. *Procedure to be followed when a high blood pressure reading is obtained* When a high blood pressure reading is obtained, the pharmacist should recommend to the patient that he should have the reading checked on two further occasions, as blood pressure can vary considerably. Preferably the repeat readings should be made on different days, with the patient as relaxed as possible during each reading. If that is not possible, the readings should be repeated at intervals of 15 minutes, during which time the patient has rested. Where the reading is high, or in a borderline case, the patient should be referred to his doctor. The pharmacist should note down each reading on the card or form which the patient can take to his doctor.

6. *Cooperation between doctors and pharmacists* Where possible, pharmacists should have preliminary talks with local doctors before using the apparatus. Any special views which the doctor may have as to the blood pressure above which the patient should be referred to him, and the procedure for repeating the measurement, could be discussed.

7. *Use of conventional sphygmomanometer apparatus* One of the main advantages of the electronic sphygmomanometer apparatus is

that it makes the detection of the sounds of blood flow in the brachial artery much easier than by use of the conventional stethoscope. Pharmacists should not, therefore, use the conventional sphygmomanometer apparatus without training and considerable experience.

Guidelines for the use of automatic apparatus for the measurement of blood pressure for use by patients

1. The apparatus It is important that the apparatus should be accurate, robust, simple to operate, and easy to clean and maintain under the conditions of use in the pharmacy. The readings of blood pressure should be clearly displayed. Manufacturers of the apparatus should be asked to produce evidence from trials that high readings of blood pressure obtained from the apparatus have subsequently been confirmed by readings taken in doctors' surgeries. If a patient is regularly checking his blood pressure during a course of treatment it may be best to suggest to him that he takes the reading on the same apparatus, thereby eliminating apparatus-to-apparatus variations. The pharmacist should ensure that the suppliers of the apparatus provide a regular service to maintain the apparatus and to check its performance.

2. Advertising the apparatus A discreet notice relating to blood pressure screening may be displayed at any pharmacy.

3. Siting the apparatus The apparatus should be sited near the dispensary so that its use can be supervised by the pharmacist. If the design of the apparatus does not ensure that the readings are visible only to the person using it, then its position should, as far as is possible, be chosen to ensure privacy.

4. Instructions for the use of the apparatus The instructions for the use of the apparatus will be provided by the manufacturer. The pharmacist should check that they are clearly displayed and always available to the user of the apparatus. The blood pressure level above which the user should consult his doctor should be given, and will probably be a diastolic pressure of 90 mmHg. Also, the instructions should draw attention to the fact that an individual's blood pressure can vary considerably and, therefore, that any high reading should be confirmed on at least two occasions. Preferably this should be on different days, with the patient as relaxed as possible during each repeat reading. If the readings cannot be taken on different days, they should be repeated on the same day at intervals of 15 minutes.

The pharmacist should also add to the manufacturer's instructions a notice to the effect that the pharmacist will advise the patient on the action he should take if he obtains a blood pressure reading above the figure given by the manufacturer.

5. *Procedure to be followed by the pharmacist when a patient draws his attention to a blood pressure reading* When a patient draws his attention to a blood pressure reading, the pharmacist should note the reading and explain the need for it to be confirmed on two further occasions, preferably on different days, with the patient in a relaxed condition. If that is not possible, the readings should be repeated at intervals of 15 minutes, during which time the patient has rested. The pharmacist should supervise the repeat readings and note them down on a card or form. As there is an increase of the normal diastolic blood pressure with age, the pharmacist should ascertain the patient's age group and only refer the patient to the doctor if the diastolic blood pressure exceeds the figure for the particular age group given in the table (shown on p. 89, under *Guidelines for the measurement of blood pressure by a pharmacist with a manually-operated electronic sphygmomanometer*). Where the reading is high, or in a borderline case, the patient should be referred to his doctor. In any conversation the pharmacist holds with the patient he must observe the usual care to ensure that he does not interfere with the patient/doctor relationship or cause undue concern. If a reading is high enough to warrant reference to a doctor, every effort should be made to reassure the patient so as to avoid precipitating a high reading at the surgery because of anxiety.

6. *Cooperation between doctors and pharmacists* Where possible, pharmacists should have preliminary talks with local doctors before installing the apparatus. Any special views which the doctor may have as to the blood pressure reading above which the patient should be referred to him, and the procedure for repeating the measurement, could be discussed.

5.9.2 Council statement on pregnancy testing in pharmacies
(Published in the *Pharmaceutical Journal*, March 14 1987)

Pregnancy testing is a professional service offered by many community pharmacists. With the increase in control on expenditure in National Health Service hospitals, it is likely that more pharmacists will wish to offer such a service. The following notes are offered as guidance.

1. Confidentiality The pharmacist must keep all information provided by the patient, and the result of the test, confidential and only disclose information with the consent of the patient.

Advice on contraception may be sought at the same time as a pregnancy test and pharmacists are reminded of the Council Statement on contraceptive advice to girls under the age of 16, first published in the *Pharmaceutical Journal* on February 15, 1986.

2. Advertising Pregnancy testing is regarded as a professional service and therefore should only be advertised in accordance with the relevant parts of the Guidance Notes contained in Section 7 of the Code of Ethics in *Medicines, ethics and practice—a guide for pharmacists*.

3. Facilities for carrying out the test A reliable method of testing should be used. It is important that care is taken to prevent contamination which can be caused by the handling of samples of urine. It should be achieved by the use of a room separate from that used for dispensing. This should be maintained in a clean and tidy condition and all working surfaces should be finished with a smooth, impervious, and washable material. Adequate lighting should be provided so that the results of the test can be read correctly. A separate sink should be provided. Procedures which ensure that no confusion occurs between samples must be devised and followed. Persons carrying out tests should wash their hands before leaving the working area. All cuts and grazes on hands or on exposed parts of the body must be covered with waterproof dressings.

4. Request for a pregnancy test A signed and dated confirmation of the request should be obtained. The form on which confirmation is obtained should state the limits of accuracy of the test. All questions relating to the test should be asked by the pharmacist and the answers recorded in writing.

5. *Records* A written record of the result of the test, together with information provided by the patient and the type of test and batch number of the test materials, should be retained by the pharmacist for at least one year. Such records must be stored safely to preserve confidentiality.

6. *Communication of the result* The result of the test should be provided in writing on a standard form. If it is necessary to convey the result by telephone, the pharmacist should be satisfied that the person requesting the information is the person who requested the test. A written confirmation of the result should be provided even when the result has been communicated by telephone. The form should be dated and give the name and address of the patient. The result should be given as positive or negative, with an explanation of such terms and the limits of accuracy of the test—for example:

The specimen provided has been tested for urinary gonadotrophin and has been found to be:

Positive   Negative

Research has shown the results of the test to be accurate in 98 per cent of all cases. A positive result indicates a probable pregnancy.

At the request of the patient, a copy of the form should be sent to her medical practitioner. Notwithstanding the result of the test, the patient should be strongly advised to consult her medical practitioner or, if she appears reluctant to do so, another source of medical advice—for example, a pregnancy advisory bureau. The pharmacist should not recommend a particular pregnancy advisory bureau but have a list available for use if the patient requests information.

5.9.3 Council guidelines on cholesterol testing
(Published in the *Pharmaceutical Journal* December 17, 1988)

Further RPSGB guidance on testing of body fluids is to be issued during 1991.
  Equipment is now available for the rapid and reliable testing of

cholesterol and triglyceride levels. This equipment is likely to be actively promoted to pharmacies, doctors' surgeries, and possibly other outlets. The Council of the Royal Pharmaceutical Society would be concerned if this service was available from premises where no professional advice was available and the public was caused much unnecessary concern.

Pharmacists are ideally placed to provide cholesterol testing in community pharmacies which are distributed throughout Great Britain. This will be a natural part of the extension of the pharmacist's role in illness prevention and health promotion. The Council has produced guidelines for pharmacists involved in blood analysis which are set out below.

1. Before providing the service, pharmacists and any other staff involved must be suitably trained in the procedures to be followed and the counselling required. They must undertake any training programme provided by the supplier to ensure competency with the equipment.

2. Pharmacists must cooperate in testing any blood serum samples provided by a central laboratory on behalf of the supplier of the equipment to ensure that the equipment is reading consistently and correctly.

3. Pharmacists must make arrangements with a local laboratory for the regular testing of blind whole blood samples to maintain confidence in the operator and the equipment.

4. Pharmacists must liaise with the local lipid clinic or other relevant clinics to ensure that they are kept abreast of developments and for advice on when to refer patients to their medical practitioners.

5. Prior to providing a service, pharmacists are advised to inform their local general medical practitioners.

6. Before undertaking a test, an explanation must be given to the patient of the procedure to be adopted and the patient's consent obtained.

7. The necessary blood sample, the test itself, and subsequent patient counselling, must be undertaken in a suitable counselling area of the pharmacy.

8. The test itself should not take place in the dispensary.

9. Suitable procedures must be adopted for the disposal of waste material, bearing in mind the risks associated with materials contaminated with blood.

10. Patients must be provided with the results in a written form. Where the results deviate from the norm, the patient's consent must be sought for this information to be sent to their general practitioner. If patients withold such agreement, they must be advised to seek medical advice, taking the written results with them.

11. Details of the result must be retained in the pharmacy.

12. Where a reading is above the optimum, in addition to counselling and advising medical treatment where appropriate, pharmacists should supply printed information leaflets which can be obtained from organizations such as the Family Heart Association, PO Box 116, Kidlington, Oxford OX5 1DT, the Health Education Authority, Hamilton House, Mableden Place, London WC1H 9TX, and the British Heart Foundation, 102, Gloucester Place, London W1H 4DH.

13. As the service is a professional service, any publicity should comply with Section 7 (vi) of the Code of Ethics contained in *Medicines, ethics and practice—a guide for pharmacists*.

Although doubts have been publicly expressed on the accuracy of some of the equipment available, the Society is not aware of any evidence for this concern. Any doubts should be allayed by the recommendation that pharmacists should cooperate in regular testing of blind serum and whole blood samples to ensure that the pharmacist has adequate experience and the equipment is reliable. Where a reading is marginally above the optimum, appropriate verbal advice should be given on diet and lifestyle, supplemented where possible by printed literature. However, where there is a need for medical intervention, the patient must be referred.

The Society's views on cholesterol screening and a copy of the guidelines have been submitted to the group set up by the Standing Medical Advisory Committee to advise the Health Minister on cholesterol screening.

6 Preventing cancer

Cancer is the second leading cause of death in the UK, accounting for around one in four of all deaths. On current rates of incidence, one in three people will develop cancer at some time in their life. Cancer is largely a disease of old age and almost three-quarters of new cases occur in people aged over 60. The degree to which cancers are preventable has been a cause of debate but it is thought that over 80 per cent of cancer is potentially avoidable. While many years of cancer research have yet to provide all the answers about the causes of cancer, the two most important risk factors are cigarette smoking and diet and, in terms of health education priorities, these are far more significant than any other risks. Pharmacists can offer advice about these and other topics related to cancer prevention.

6.1 Mortality from cancer

While research has improved the prognosis for many cancers, particularly childhood cancers such as leukaemia, some of the commoner types are usually too advanced for curative treatment by the time they can be diagnosed. Thus, the main way to improve survival is by strategies aimed at prevention and early detection, as well as by developing better therapies. In 1988, 162 000 men and women died from cancer in the United Kingdom; Table 6.1 shows the cancers which cause the most deaths in men and women separately. Cancer was the cause of a quarter of all deaths in the UK in 1988.

Pharmacists are asked for advice about a wide range of symptoms and health matters. We will go on to consider the different types of cancer, the factors which are known to be involved in their development, and the potential role of the pharmacist in their detection and prevention.

Table 6.1 Deaths from cancer in the UK in 1988

Men			*Women*		
Lung	27 970	(33%)	Breast	15 300	(20%)
Prostate	8230	(10%)	Lung	12 260	(16%)
Stomach	6320	(7%)	Colon	7110	(9%)
Colon	5860	(7%)	Stomach	4290	(6%)
Bladder	3670	(4%)	Ovary	4280	(5%)
Rectum	3570	(4%)	Pancreas	3510	(5%)
Oesophagus	3360	(4%)	Rectum	2920	(4%)
Pancreas	3280	(4%)	Oesophagus	2230	(3%)
Leukaemia	2170	(3%)	Cervix	2170	(3%)
Brain	1660	(2%)	Leukaemia	1910	(2%)
Others		(22%)	Others		(27%)

(Source: Cancer Research Campaign Statistics 1990)

6.2 Lung cancer

This is by far the leading cause of cancer deaths and almost entirely preventable—over 90 per cent of all lung cancer mortality is attributable to cigarette smoking. In 1988 lung cancer was responsible for 33 per cent of all male and 16 per cent of all female deaths from cancer. Among men the rates of lung cancer have been falling since the 1960s but among women the opposite has occurred. The death rates among women have accelerated to the extent that lung cancer overtook breast cancer as the leading cause of cancer death in Scottish women in 1987, and the same is likely to occur for England and Wales.

Historically, at the time of the First World War many men took up smoking, but the increase in smoking among women did not occur until during and after the Second World War. Current concern is that much of the advertising for cigarettes is aimed at women, and at young women in particular. Levels of smoking among schoolchildren in the UK show that more teenage girls are beginning to smoke than are teenage boys.

For the pharmacist, offering advice on smoking cessation is the most effective way of preventing lung cancer. Thought can be given to directing material at the mothers of teenage children, since these women frequently visit community pharmacies. The pharmacist can, therefore, be a source of advice and support for smokers and other members of their families. Advice on stopping smoking can be found in Chapter 7 (p. 115).

Community pharmacists are frequently asked to respond to symptoms, and a persistent unexplained cough (particularly if associated with blood in sputum and any degree of breathing difficulty) will always be a cause for immediate referral to the customer's GP. The problem among smokers is of course that, since many have a continual cough, the early symptoms of lung cancer may be undetected. The incidence of lung cancer rises steeply with increasing age and pharmacists should be aware of chronic cough in an older person, particularly a non-smoker. For smokers, where the ubiquitous 'smoker's cough' may be present, other symptoms such as pain on coughing, blood in the sputum and unexplained weight loss are further indicators of serious pathology. Unexpected and unexplained weight loss in someone middle-aged or older is a strong indication of serious disease, especially cancer.

6.3 Large bowel (colorectal) cancer

This is the second leading cause of cancer deaths in both men and women and now claims almost 20 000 lives a year in the United Kingdom. If detected in the early stages the prognosis is promising, and here pharmacists can be alert for signs and symptoms which suggest the possibility of bowel cancer.

Although worldwide research points to the importance of diet in connection with bowel cancer, the evidence about specific items of diet is still unclear. However, overall dietary recommendations can be made because some of the evidence supports them and the kind of diet recommended is likely to be beneficial for general health.

Many studies have shown an association between bowel cancer and a diet that is high in fat, high in red meat consumption, and low in fibre. These studies have dealt with whole populations and the evidence from individual case studies is less convincing. It seems sensible to reduce the intake of dietary fat because there is still a possibility that it may promote some cancers and a low-fat diet may also reduce the risk of heart disease. A level of fat intake of not more than 30 per cent of total calories is generally recommended.

Again, there is a lack of consistency in the evidence about diets which protect against bowel cancer. Dietary fibre has for some time been considered an important ingredient of a healthy diet, but confusion has arisen because there are many different types of 'fibre' (non-starch polysaccharides) and they differ in their effects. Soluble fibre may help to lower serum cholesterol concentration, non-soluble fibres may affect bowel movement, acting as a laxative. People who consume a diet which is low in fibre tend to be constipated, so that food stays in the gut for far longer than when a high-fibre diet is eaten. This increased transit time of food associated with a low-fibre diet is thought to expose the wall of the gut to carcinogenic substances in foods and to allow the conversion of some substances into more harmful forms. These facts strengthen the case for the pharmacist to offer dietary advice to those who are constipated (for further details, see p. 143 of Chapter 9). If fibre has a protective effect, it seems more likely that it is the specific components of fibre, rather than total consumption, that are beneficial.

The main foods which provide dietary fibre are fruits, vegetables, grains, and cereals. These also contain various vitamins and minerals that may help protect against cancer. Research has shown that foods high in betacarotene (converted to vitamin A in the body), vitamin C, and vitamin E may all offer some protection. Adequate supplies of vitamins can be derived from a diet containing plenty of vegetables, salads, and fruit, and the benefits of supplements are uncertain. The mineral selenium, which seems to offer some protection, can be toxic when taken at higher than recommended doses as a supplement.

Risk factors for bowel cancer include a family history of bowel cancer, or of polyps in the bowel (polyposis), or a history of inflammatory bowel disease.

Bowel cancer is rare in the under-50s and thus it is the older age group who are most at risk. The pharmacist should be particularly alert for symptoms which have occurred over a long period of time or which have gradually worsened in this age group. A prolonged and unexplained change in bowel habit lasting over two weeks, particularly if accompanied by rectal bleeding, is an indication for referral. Unexplained weight loss is a further indicator of serious pathology.

A possible role for pharmacists in the future will be in the sale of screening tests for bowel cancer. Such tests are widely available in the United States and are being evaluated in the United Kingdom.

They aim to detect small amounts of blood in the stools (occult blood). The presence of blood in the stools can be a sign of cancer although it can also occur in other, benign conditions. The efficacy of these tests is not yet established and the rate of false positive results has so far prevented their widespread use in screening. Several types of kits for haemoccult testing are being investigated. If screening tests are to be made available through pharmacies, pharmacists will need additional training in the scientific basis for the tests, and thus the way in which false positive results can be the consequence of dietary intake and drugs, so that appropriate advice can be given. As for any other type of screening, careful attention and thought must be paid to the ethical aspects of the procedure and to the pharmacist's duty of care in possessing the appropriate and current skills and knowledge in relation to the test (see Chapter 5, p. 85).

6.4 Breast cancer

Some 15 000 women die from breast cancer each year in the UK and there are over 25 000 new cases. Breast cancer is rare in men, with around 170 new cases and 100 deaths annually. The high level of deaths from breast cancer can only be reduced by improving methods of detecting the disease and treating it at an early stage. After a careful assessment of the risks and benefits of screening, a decision was taken to set up a national programme in the UK using mammography—a form of X-ray investigation. Mammography trials in New York and Sweden showed reductions in mortality of up to 30 per cent. Routine screening by mammography is now being offered to all women aged between 50 and 64 and repeated every three years. The time interval is being kept under review. Women aged 65 and over may be screened on request. The screening is less effective in women under 50, but further research will be carried out on this issue.

While women are probably unlikely to consult their pharmacist about breast symptoms rather than their GP, there is nevertheless an important role for the pharmacist in stocking leaflets about self-examination of the breasts. In addition, the pharmacist can be aware of local testing facilities and of the details of mammography if questions about the procedure should be raised, which is possible in the essentially informal atmosphere of the pharmacy, where women may express their fears and concerns.

There is evidence that a high-fat diet may increase the risk of breast cancer, by promoting cancer rather than initiating it. Which components of fat are important is still uncertain. Excessive fat intake, resulting in obesity, has been linked with increased risk of breast cancer, though more in post-menopausal than in younger women. Recently, there have been several 'scares' about use of the combined oral contraceptive pill and the risk of breast cancer. The results of studies have been conflicting. The potential benefits and drawbacks of the combined oral contraceptive pill are discussed further in Chapter 11 (see p. 164). The possibility of a small increase in risk of breast cancer from hormone replacement therapy (HRT) has also been raised. In the case of HRT the beneficial protective effects against cardiovascular disease and osteoporosis must be set against the possible increased risk from breast cancer.

6.5 Cervical cancer

In 1988, 2170 women died from cervical cancer in the United Kingdom. A national screening programme is in operation, using the smear test to facilitate early detection, since at the early stages the disease is asymptomatic. Survival rates are very good for women whose cancer is treated early. Screening is intended to reduce incidence and mortality from cervical cancer by detecting and treating conditions that might otherwise develop into cancer. To ensure the good results that have been seen in countries with well-organized screening programmes, it is essential to have a high participation rate and adequate follow-up after each smear test.

Over the last ten to fifteen years there has been an increase in mortality in younger women (those aged from 25–34) and a decrease in women aged 45 and over. More than 80 per cent of invasive disease is, however, found in women aged over 35, and the great majority of these have never been screened. Women aged 20–64 should have a smear test every three years. The problems of ensuring a high uptake of cervical cancer screening are particularly acute in inner city and deprived areas and among older women—to date the screening programme has failed to reach those most at risk.

The pharmacist has an important role in stocking literature about screening for cervical cancer and in encouraging its uptake.

Evidence from research suggests that cervical cancer may be a preventable disease which is caused by a sexually-transmitted agent, possibly a genital wart virus. Known risks are early age of first intercourse and multiple sexual partners. A woman's risk is increased by the number of sexual contacts her male partner has had. Smoking appears to increase susceptibility to the disease. Barrier methods of contraception can reduce the risk, and it is thought that, among women who take oral contraceptive pills, the higher rate of cervical cancer may be due to the lack of barrier protection against the sexually-transmitted agent. While there is a possibility that the pill itself may increase the risk of cancer, this has not been proved. Increasing numbers of young women aged between 25 and 34 are dying from cervical cancer although the total number of deaths in this age group is still small (110 per annum). It is thought that changes in sexual behaviour and contraception practices in the last two decades have led to this increase. For the pharmacist, the availability of leaflets on the choice of contraception, on local family planning clinics and contraceptive advice, and on screening for cervical cancer is important in making sure that information gets across to women.

6.6 Skin cancer

The commoner types of skin cancer occur mainly in the elderly and account for some 10 per cent of all cancers in this country. These cancers are seldom fatal, since they very rarely metastasize and can be cured. Basal cell carcinoma (rodent ulcer) occurs mainly on the head or neck. The less common squamous cell carcinomas may also present as ulcers.

A far rarer type of skin cancer, malignant melanoma, accounts for about 1 per cent of all cancer cases but causes over 1100 deaths each year. The chances of cure are very good if treatment can be carried out at an early stage of the melanoma's development, before it has begun to spread. It is therefore essential to improve detection of the early signs of malignant melanoma and to educate people about protecting their skin, and their children's, so as to reduce the risk of developing this dangerous disease.

Excessive exposure to the sun, particularly over short periods of time, and bad sunburn, in childhood as well as in adulthood, is known to be associated with an increased risk of malignant melanoma. Thus, as the number of people taking holidays in hot countries has increased, so has the incidence of melanoma. There were 2626 new cases of malignant melanoma in 1984, two-thirds of which were in women, compared with 1735 in 1974.

There are several types of malignant melanoma, the commonest of which is superficial spreading melanoma. This may start from a mole or freckle and is often on the lower leg in women and on the back in men. Nodular melanomas account for about one-quarter of all melanomas and are commoner in men, often occurring on the trunk. They grow relatively rapidly and may bleed at a fairly early stage. Then there is the rather slow-growing type, often found in people over 60, frequently on the cheek. A fourth type of melanoma can arise in and around the nail bed, especially on the big toe.

In around one-third of cases the melanoma develops from a pre-existing mole, and it is therefore important for the public to be on the lookout for any potentially sinister changes. The following signs have been associated with melanoma:

Major skin signs for referral to the doctor:

1. Is an existing mole getting larger or a new one growing? After puberty moles usually do not grow.

2. Does it have a ragged outline? Ordinary moles are smooth and have a regular shape.

3. Does it have a mixture of different shades of brown and black? Ordinary moles may be quite dark brown or black but are all one shade.

Any of these may also be present in a melanoma:

4. Is it bigger than the blunt end of a pencil? Most normal moles are smaller than this.

5. Is the mole inflamed or does it have a reddish edge? An ordinary one is not inflamed.

6. Is it bleeding, oozing, or crusting? Ordinary moles do not do this.

7. Is there a change in sensation, like a mild itch? An ordinary mole
   is not usually itchy or painful.

(From the Cancer Research Campaign, 'Be a Mole Watcher')

Any pharmacy customer who describes such changes—usually
at least two or three signs will be present—should be referred
immediately to their GP.

Melanoma is one of the few cancers to have a significant impact
on young adults, although it is extremely rare in childhood. One
in five of those who develop melanoma are aged under forty
(compared with 4 per cent for all cancers). The prognosis and survival of those patients treated before the cancer has metastasized
are very good. Outlook also depends on the thickness of the cancer
(Breslow thickness)—there is very good survival for those with
'thin' tumours.

Those most at risk are fair-skinned, fair- or red-haired, with light-
coloured eyes, who never tan or burn before they tan. Evidence
suggests that damage to the skin caused by sunburn, even in
childhood years, can increase later risk of melanoma. Also at risk
are those with a large number of ordinary moles—over 60 in young
people, over 50 in older people. Unusual moles (large, irregular,
and multicoloured) are a risk factor. Another is a family history of
melanoma, or having previously had a melanoma.

The classification of skin types and appropriate sun-protection
factors is shown in Table 6.2 below.

Table 6.2 Skin types and recommended sun protection factors (SPF)

Skin type	Tanning ability	Recommended SPF
Type 1	White skin. Never tans, always burns.	10–15
Type 2	White skin. Burns initially, tans with difficulty.	8–9
Type 3	White skin. Tans easily, burns rarely.	6–7
Type 4	White skin. Never burns, always tans.	4–5
Type 5	Brown skin (Asian and mongoloid).	2–3
Type 6	Black skin (Afro-Caribbean).	None

Generally, the best advice to minimize the risk of skin cancer is to spend a minimum of time in the sun, wear light protective clothing, and avoid exposure during the middle of the day. However, pharmacists will be well aware that many of their customers will wish to go on gaining a 'healthy' tan while on holiday. Advice can be offered about the most appropriate use of sunscreens and an explanation can be given about the potential risks. Information given to parents may help to change attitudes towards sunbathing where children may be at risk. Practical advice to help understanding of the SPF system is always useful. Many people continue to use either no sunscreen or one which gives insufficient protection. The SPF represents the time taken to produce erythema in skin covered with the sun-screen compared with unprotected skin. Thus, if someone normally burned in the sun after 30 minutes, wearing a sunscreen of SPF 10 would allow a total exposure time of up to 30 × 10 (300) minutes. UVB rays promote tanning and burn unprotected skin rapidly, while UVA rays promote tanning with less risk of burning. The SPF relates only to protection against UVB rays, since it is they that are responsible for sunburn. However, sunscreens should be recommended which contain a mix of agents which screen both UVA and UVB sunlight. Recent evidence suggests that protection against both types of rays is important. When high SPF sunscreens which offer protection predominantly against UVB light are worn, people may spend many hours in the sun with substantial exposure to UVA radiation. The risk is that the long-term effects of high doses of UVA are unknown. Accelerated ageing effects on the skin are likely to result from overexposure to UVA. For similar reasons, doctors advise against the use of sunbeds. Although they have not been proved to cause skin cancer, they do allow the skin to be damaged and 'age'. The tan acquired from a sunbed gives little protection against the sun.

Those pharmacy customers who ask advice about the choice of sunscreen for a summer or winter holiday should be questioned about their history of tanning and burning which, together with an assessment of skin type, can be used as the basis for a recommendation. Parents should use products with a high SPF on their children's skin, since there is evidence that sunburn in childhood can increase the likelihood of malignant melanoma in later life. For those who wish to tan, current advice is that spending short periods of time in the sun with a sunscreen of relatively low SPF may be better than long periods with a high SPF. Naturally, care must still be taken to avoid burning.

Pharmacists can also offer simple practical advice to prevent sunburn. Sunbathing between 10 am and 3 pm coincides with the period when the most ultraviolet energy is striking the earth. The midday sun is the strongest of all and most likely to burn, so sunbathing times should be carefully planned. One simple tip is that when the person's shadow is at its shortest, the sun is overhead, and its rays at their strongest. The closer the length of the shadow to the person's actual height, the less strong the sun's rays. At high altitudes less of the sun's energy is filtered out, so skin damage is more likely. Particular care should be taken when swimming—sun penetrates water. Wearing a shirt can prevent the shoulders and back from burning. The wearing of a hat is to be encouraged and is of particular importance for children.

6.7 The European 10-Point cancer code

We have considered some of the commonly-occurring cancers and ways in which pharmacists might offer advice to their customers. In the campaign 'Europe Against Cancer', health educators throughout Europe are attempting to educate the public about ways in

---

The European 10-Point cancer code

1. Stop smoking
2. Stay within safe alcohol limits
3. Avoid being overweight
4. Take care in the sun
5. Observe health and safety regulations at work
6. Cut down on fatty foods
7. Eat plenty of fresh fruit and vegetables and other foods containing fibre
8. See your doctor if there is any unexplained change in your normal health which lasts longer than two weeks (e.g. change in bowel habit)
9. and 10. (For women) Have a regular cervical smear test and examine your breasts each month

---

which the risk of cancer might be reduced, and about the early warning signs and symptoms of cancer. The European Cancer Code is summarized below, and pharmacists can use this as a reference point for advice-giving.

This code aims to reduce deaths from cancer in Europe by 1500 annually by the year 2000 and is publicized by European countries. The code is based on existing knowledge about prevention and early detection of cancer.

7 Smoking

One third of all adults smoke and studies have shown that 60–70 per cent of these would like to stop. There is an important role for pharmacists in giving advice about how to stop smoking and in stocking leaflets and information about smoking cessation. While most ex-smokers stopped without using any form of medication, many community pharmacies stock anti-smoking products, and later in this chapter we will discuss their pharmacological effects and role in anti-smoking advice. Pharmacists could be more pro-active rather than reactive in the area of smoking cessation, giving advice opportunistically, as we shall show.

7.1 Epidemiology

During the early 1970s, half of all adults in the UK smoked cigarettes—this percentage has now fallen to one-third. Until recently the decrease was continuous and steady, and total cigarette sales have dropped by nearly one-third over the past decade.

Tobacco was introduced into England at the time of King James I and here, as in other countries, strenuous efforts were made to stamp out this 'noxious weed'. The smoking habit nevertheless became more common during the second half of the nineteenth century. Cigarette smoking began in the higher social classes and mostly among men, and around 1900 it was still uncommon to see people smoking cigarettes in public. The fashion then spread to other social classes, partly because cigarettes were tax-free to those in the trenches during the First World War. Cigarette smoking among women was established later, after the Second World War, and it became more socially accepted for women to smoke.

The social change now taking place is in the reverse order. Men in higher social groups are discarding the habit and are being followed more slowly by manual workers and by women, in both of whom the rate of stopping is lower. In the early 1950s almost 70 per cent of men and 40 per cent of women smoked—in 1988 the corresponding figures were 33 per cent men and 30 per cent women, with a higher percentage in socioeconomic groups IIIM, IV, and V (see Table 7.1). Concern has been expressed about the numbers of young people who start to smoke. In 1989 surveys showed that 17 per cent of 15-year-old boys and 24 per cent of 15-year-old girls smoke regularly. Health educators have tried for many years to prevent young people from starting to smoke. Generally, smoking habits become established during adolescence, and it is unusual for people to start to smoke after the age of 20. Research has shown that children are more likely to smoke if one or both of their parents do so. Peer group pressure is an important factor, and the image of

Table 7.1 Prevalence of cigarette smoking by sex and socioeconomic group in Great Britain: 1972–84. Persons aged 16 and over†

Socioeconomic group	Percentage smoking cigarettes								
	1972	1974	1976	1978	1980	1982	1984	1986	1988
MEN									
Professional	33	29	25	25	21	20	17	18	16
Employers and managers	44	46	38	37	35	29	29	28	26
Intermediate and junior non-manual	45	45	40	38	35	30	30	28	25
Skilled manual and own account non-professional	57	56	51	49	48	42	40	40	39
Semi-skilled manual and personal service	57	56	53	53	49	47	45	43	40
Unskilled manual	64	61	58	60	57	49	49	43	43
All aged 16 and over†	52	51	46	45	42	38	36	35	33
WOMEN									
Professional	33	25	28	23	21	21	15	19	17
Employers and managers	38	38	35	33	33	29	29	27	26
Intermediate and junior non-manual	38	38	36	33	34	30	28	27	27
Skilled manual and own account non-professional	47	46	42	42	43	39	37	36	35
Semi-skilled manual and personal service	42	43	41	41	39	36	37	35	37
Unskilled manual	42	43	38	41	41	41	36	33	39
All aged 16 and over†	42	41	38	37	37	33	32	31	30

† Aged 15 and over in 1972.
(Source: Office of population censuses and surveys)

smoking is still sometimes seen as a rebellious and anti-establishment gesture by children.

7.1.1 How smoking damages health

Tobacco smoke contains over 3900 chemical constituents and the damaging constituents of cigarettes include carbon monoxide, nicotine, and tar. Carbon monoxide combines with haemoglobin in the blood to form carboxyhaemoglobin, which restricts the uptake of oxygen. This reaction is irreversible and thus the oxygen-carrying capacity of the blood is reduced in smokers, putting additional strain on the heart. Nicotine stimulates the heart, increasing its rate and adding to its workload. The vasoconstriction caused by nicotine, together with poor peripheral oxygenation, can damage the circulation to the extent that amputation of part of the lower leg has to be performed. Tar contains carcinogenic substances and is responsible for causing lung cancer. Tar is a complex mixture of hundreds of chemicals, many of which have been shown to cause cancer in laboratory animals. Lower tar cigarettes are associated with a lower risk of lung cancer but an identical risk of heart disease as from standard cigarettes. Herbal cigarettes are available and, in our increasingly health-conscious society, are sometimes seen as a 'healthier' alternative. That is not the case—while nicotine will not be present, the problems of habituation, carbon monoxide, tar, and the irritant effects of smoke on the lungs, still occur.

7.2 Health risks from smoking

The dangers of smoking cigarettes are well-known and the fact that they are a major cause of lung and other cancers, and of coronary heart disease, is also well-established. These hazards will be considered in turn.

7.2.1 Smoking and cancer

Lung cancer is the most common form of the disease for men and accounts for one-third of total cancer deaths. For women, the rates doubled between 1963 and 1983, and in Scotland lung cancer overtook breast cancer as the leading cause of cancer mortality amongst women in 1987. Lung cancer rates in the UK are falling steadily but remain amongst the highest in the world.

While lung cancer is the greatest concern (over 90 per cent of lung cancer deaths are attributable to cigarette smoking), smoking increases the risk of other cancers, including those of the mouth, larynx, oesophagus, and bladder. The reduction of tar levels of cigarettes and the introduction of filters has also played a part in reducing lung cancer rates.

7.2.2 Smoking and heart disease

Smoking is implicated in the incidence of coronary heart disease and epidemiological studies demonstrate that it is one of the most important risk factors. The risk of developing heart disease is three times greater for those smoking over 30 cigarettes a day than for non-smokers. The precise mechanism by which smoking causes heart disease is unclear but would seem to be related to one of the constituents of tobacco being a major causative influence in the development of atherosclerosis. Smoking causes a reduction in HDL cholesterol and affects the haemostatic system by decreasing platelet survival time and increasing platelet stickiness and tendency to aggregate.

Studies have shown a consistent gradient in the reduction in risk for coronary heart disease as the time since stopping smoking increases. This benefit is seen for all age groups and for both heavy and light smokers. It is therefore worthwhile emphasizing to would-be ex-smokers that stopping smoking is worthwhile—it is not the case that all the damage has already been done.

7.2.3 Smoking and respiratory disease

Cigarette smoking is one of the major causes of chronic obstructive airways disease. Morbidity and mortality from chronic bronchitis and emphysema are substantially higher in smokers than in non-smokers. In addition, cigarette smokers of all ages have more chest illnesses than do non-smokers—cough and recurrent chest-infections result in considerable morbidity and absenteeism from work. Although some smokers die from their obstructive airways disease, stopping smoking reduces the risk of dying from this cause.

In the pharmacy, advice about treatment for coughs is often

sought by patients with chronic bronchitis as a result of cigarette smoking. Many community pharmacists offer a service of delivering oxygen cylinders to those patients whose lung disease has progressed to emphysema, where large pockets in the lungs prevent efficient gaseous exchange. Many of these patients have reached the stage where they are unable to function without medicinal oxygen. The mobility of such patients is severely restricted, and in the later stages of emphysema the patient may be completely housebound and reliant on the pharmacist's delivery of oxygen and medication.

7.2.4 Smoking and pregnancy

Smoking by pregnant women has been shown to lead to an increased risk for low birth weight. Two factors contribute to this risk—retardation of intra-uterine growth and an increased risk of premature birth. The fetus obtains less oxygen because blood levels of carbon monoxide and carbon dioxide are higher in pregnant women who smoke.

7.2.5 Passive smoking

There is increasing evidence from research to show that passive smoking has adverse effects on health, particularly that of babies and young children whose parents smoke. Such children have been shown to suffer from more respiratory problems than do the offspring of non-smokers. For asthmatic patients, working or living with someone who smokes will exacerbate the condition. Epidemiological studies have shown that non-smoking spouses and partners of smokers have a higher risk of lung cancer as a result of passive smoking. Smoking in the workplace has also become an important health and safety issue as a result of the growing body of evidence about the health risks of passive smoking.

7.3 Why have people stopped smoking?

Since the late 1960s, in the UK, as in almost all advanced industrial nations, the proportion of the population who smoke has gradually fallen. Three major issues have contributed to this reduction—price, public education, and the social environment. We will go on to consider each of these.

7.3.1 Cigarette prices and consumption

Studies in several countries have shown that market demand for cigarettes varies inversely with their price—that is, that cigarette consumption falls when prices rise and vice versa. Price has been shown to be an important determinant of smoking levels.

Studies which have examined the impact of pricing policy on cigarette consumption have used the *real* costs of cigarettes as their baseline. The real price is the current price divided by the retail price index. Inflation can have a major effect on the real price of cigarettes because if cigarette taxation is not increased in line with inflation, the real price of cigarettes falls. Estimates of the influence of price on consumption state that, for every 1 per cent increase in price, consumption may fall by 0.5 per cent.

Most smokers acknowledge a price ceiling beyond which they would have, or would choose, to give up. The continued pressure to increase the tax on tobacco products by a rate in excess of inflation is based on the price sensitivity of the tobacco market. Figures for the UK from 1971–85 show clearly that smoking increased when tax increases failed to keep up with inflation. Smoking fell when the real price of cigarettes increased in the mid-1970s and during the 1980s.

Different sections of the community are likely to respond to price changes in different ways. Research suggests that the price of cigarettes is a strong determinant of teenage smoking and that price increases would have a strong deterrent effect for this group. Smoking is a major contributor to the health differentials between lower and higher socioeconomic groups. There is evidence to show that those in lower income groups are more sensitive to cigarette price changes, smoking less when cigarettes become more expensive and more when they become cheaper. Falls in the price of cigarettes effectively negate the work of health educators. It has been argued that large decreases in total tobacco consumption will only happen when 'health education is supported by a price policy consistent with health objectives'.

7.3.2 Public education

Publication of anti-smoking reports by the Royal College of Physicians in 1962 and 1971 was followed by a reduction in smoking. In the United Kingdom, before the publication of these and other early reports which identified the health risks of smoking, there was little difference in smoking rates between socioeconomic groups. By 1988 though, 43 per cent of unskilled working class men (social class V) smoked cigarettes while only 16 per cent of professional men (social class I) did so.

Extensive health education campaigns and activities initiated both by government bodies such as the Health Education Authority and by pressure groups like Action on Smoking and Health (ASH) have publicized the health risks of smoking to a mass audience. The correlation between lung cancer and smoking is solidly established both in clinical trials and animal experiments. This message appears to have been widely received by the public, many of whom now know of the association between smoking and lung cancer. The connection between smoking and coronary heart disease is less well-known among members of the public, although more smokers are likely to die prematurely of heart disease than of lung cancer.

Advertising of cigarettes has been banned on British television, and the Health Education Authority has funded many anti-smoking drives and has supported specific initiatives such as 'National No Smoking Day'. However, the UK can be criticized for not going as far as other countries who have banned all forms of tobacco advertising and require firmer and more explicit health warnings to be printed on every cigarette packet. There is a voluntary agreement between tobacco manufacturers and government whereby the nature and extent of advertising, and the wording of warning statements on cigarette packaging, are negotiated rather than stated in legislation. This ambivalence must be at least partly due to a reluctance to lose tax revenues from tobacco, which makes successive governments hesitate to price cigarettes as luxuries. The success (or otherwise) of the voluntary agreement has been a matter for debate. Sponsorship of televised sporting events is one way in which tobacco companies overcome the ban on television advertising of cigarettes. Tobacco advertising promotes the idea that smoking is acceptable, desirable, and glamorous, and undermines the credibility of health education messages.

7.3.3 The social environment

Social pressures to stop smoking appear to be growing. Local and national pressure groups have mounted concerted and effective campaigns to have smoking curtailed. Many theatres, cinemas, and restaurants now operate no-smoking policies or offer non-smoking seating areas and these are increasingly accepted as the norm. Some airlines have banned smoking on their flights. Since the majority of workers are now non-smokers, no-smoking policies in the work-place are increasingly being implemented with either a ban on smoking or designated areas and time periods for smoking. Where companies develop no-smoking policies, counselling and advice is usually offered to members of staff to help them to stop smoking. The Royal Pharmaceutical Society of Great Britain instituted a total ban on smoking in its premises from 1 January 1991.

Even smokers think that smoking should be banned in public places—a quarter of smokers say they would favour a ban in all public places, over 40 per cent on public transport, in restaurants, and cinemas, and over 70 per cent in shops.

If this momentum to stop smoking continues, and if we as pharmacists play our part in helping people to 'kick the habit', then by the end of this century it may be as unusual to see someone smoking in public as it was at the beginning of it.

7.4 Advice on how to stop smoking

There are now 10 million ex-smokers in the UK. While stopping is very difficult for some, many people stop with relative lack of difficulty. More than half the ex-smokers interviewed in a major survey said they had not found it difficult to stop. A third said they sometimes missed smoking but 86 per cent said they thought they were unlikely to start again.

Where the pharmacist has previously smoked, that personal ex-perience may be valuable in giving advice. Most people need more than one attempt to stop smoking and it has been shown that many succeed even after many failed attempts. It is important to tell the customer this so that there is no sense of failure after the first try.

The majority of ex-smokers stop without taking any medication, and thus the giving of advice about how to stop smoking need not be routinely related to the use of anti-smoking products. Pharmacy undergraduates learn predominantly about disease states and their treatment using drugs. In health education advice, the emphasis is on helping people to make choices and changing their behaviour rather than on medicine taking.

All smokers know that smoking is bad for them, most know it causes lung cancer, and an increasing number know of other health hazards. Smokers are told constantly by the media and others that smoking is a dirty and antisocial habit; accordingly, pharmacists do not need to repeat any of this information. Health education research has shown clearly that stressing health risks may not always be the most effective way to achieve the behaviour change sought. Some smokers have heard so often about the health risks from smoking that they believe that, for them, the damage is already done and so it is not worth stopping. Pharmacists have an important role in explaining that the health risks can still be reduced, stressing the benefits of stopping.

An appropriate response to a request from somebody who wishes to stop smoking would be to welcome that decision and to stress the main benefits of stopping, which include:

- saving money;
- feeling cleaner and fresher;
- better health.

In order to create an environment where people are likely to seek advice, we think that the pharmacy should be a 'no-smoking' area with signs and stickers to that effect, that the pharmacy should have signs inviting people to ask for advice about stopping smoking, and should have a display of leaflets and information material. Whilst there are no hard and fast rules, the Health Education Authority's advice on how to stop is as follows:

1. *Pick a day to stop—identify an actual date.* The two main reasons for this action are the psychological effect of planning to stop smoking after a specific time and the practical advantage of not choosing a day to stop when the customer is likely to be under stress—for example, moving house or having a job interview. The Health Education Authority suggests that a time be chosen when stress is likely to be minimal.

2. *Tell all your friends and relatives.* The reason for this is to enlist moral support both from friends and family members.

3. *Throw away the paraphernalia of smoking, i.e. cigarettes, matches, and ashtrays.* There are two reasons for this: firstly, the psychological result of discarding the materials of smoking; and secondly the practical result of not having cigarettes around when the urge to smoke might be there.

4. *Stop and stay stopped.*

The pharmacist can add a *fifth* point, which is to invite the customer to return to the pharmacy and tell the pharmacist how he or she has got on. If the person who returns has started to smoke again, the pharmacist can be supportive and suggest choosing another day and trying again. After more than one unsuccessful attempt, the pharmacist might consider referral to the doctor or to an anti-smoking clinic run by the local health authority (if there is such a clinic locally). The Quitline telephone number may be used to obtain details of anti-smoking clinics (071 323 0505).

Where the person has stopped for a short period of time they may feel that they have totally succeeded; the pharmacist can then advise that a further target of several weeks should be set because the difficulty will be to get through stressful periods without restarting. Increasing confidence in eventual success can sustain the ex-smoker, and support is important here.

People who want to stop smoking often ask the pharmacist's advice about which medicines they can take to help them stop. These will now be considered.

7.4.1 Over-the-counter anti-smoking products

Whilst most people successfully stop smoking without taking any product, for some people the benefit of initially exchanging one habit for another is useful, and a belief that an over-the-counter product can help may be strong. There is thus a psychological/placebo effect which may be valuable. It is important that customers' expectations of anti-smoking products should not be too high. The products should be regarded only as behaviour substitutes which will finally have to be discontinued. Anti-smoking products include:

- lozenges containing extract of nicotine ('Resolution', 'Stoppers', 'Stubit');

- 'Nicorette' chewing gum—which contains nicotine and is available on private prescription and over the counter;

- 'Nicobrevin' (menthyl valerianate + quinine);

- silver acetate chewing gum ('Tabmint').

Products containing nicotine

Research has shown that anti-smoking lozenges containing nicotine provide a significant dose of the drug. Such lozenges are manufactured as confectionery items and are widely available under the brand names 'Resolution' and 'Stoppers' (0.5 mg nicotine) and 'Stubits' (1.1 mg nicotine). As a nicotine substitute these products may help some smokers and should be dissolved slowly in the mouth.

Nicotine chewing gum ('Nicorette') is available in 2 mg and 4 mg strengths and is an anti-smoking product which has been shown to be successful as an additional aid in helping smokers to stop. Despite attempts to make the product prescribable on the National Health Service, it remains available only on private prescription. Many pharmacists have argued that they should be able to sell Nicorette over the counter and that the transfer of this product from the prescription-only list could be to patients' benefit. In fact 'Nicorette' 2 mg is likely to move from POM to P in 1991. As we have said, anti-smoking products may substitute one dependence for another, and some pharmacists occasionally report customers who have stopped smoking but are now addicted to 'Nicorette'. Such addiction, while unfortunate, is undoubtedly a lesser risk to health than is cigarette smoking.

For 'Nicorette' to be successful, a clear explanation must be given about its use. Nicotine is destroyed in the stomach and the product will only work if the nicotine is absorbed sublingually. The gum should therefore not be chewed in the manner of a traditional chewing gum, where the saliva is swallowed. Instead, a stick of 'Nicorette' should be chewed 6–10 times, then 'parked' against the gum in a corner of the mouth to allow absorption of the drug through the buccal mucosa. A stick of gum should be chewed whenever the desire to smoke occurs and many people require around ten pieces of 2 mg gum each day initially. After up to three months use, 'Nicorette' should be gradually withdrawn. Side-effects include soreness of the mouth and throat, hiccuping, indigestion, and heartburn. Excessive consumption can cause nausea, faintness, and headaches. It is essential that a clear explanation of use is given when the gum is supplied by the pharmacist. Supportive advice and an invitation to return to the pharmacy to discuss progress are important.

Menthyl valerianate and quinine ('Nicobrevin')

This product is promoted by the manufacturers on the basis that the valerianate provides a relaxing effect and the quinine content provides relief from nicotine withdrawal symptoms. One clinical trial has been performed with the product which appeared to show some benefit. The evidence is less clear than for nicotine chewing gum.

Silver acetate gum ('Tabmint')

This gum induces an unpleasant taste when a cigarette is subsequently smoked and can therefore be regarded as a form of aversion therapy. There have been no scientific trials of its effectiveness.

Simple sugar-free confectionery chewing gum may be helpful as a habit substitute for some people.

7.4.2 Acupuncture and hypnotherapy

Some smokers have found these methods to be helpful in giving up smoking. The pharmacist might consider keeping details of local availability of these services should patients request information about them. A list of medically-qualified hypnotists can be obtained from The British Society of Medical and Dental Hypnosis (see Appendix 2). A list of medically-qualified acupuncturists is available from the British Medical Acupuncture Society (see Appendix 2).

7.5 Case studies

'I want to stop smoking—what can I take?'

A young man aged about twenty has come into the pharmacy and asked for advice. The pharmacist should recognize that the customer has already decided that he wants to stop smoking. Research has shown that self-motivation to stop is essential for success. Where the customer says: 'My family/doctor/friend says I should stop', a strong indication is being given that the person concerned has no real wish to do so, and any advice which is given is less likely to succeed.

The pharmacist can welcome the decision to stop and make a general statement about the benefits of stopping. The customer in this case had asked which products were available to help him stop smoking. Before considering any product recommendation the pharmacist would normally ask a series of questions to clarify the symptoms and appropriateness of medication. There are arguments for and against asking questions about details of the person's smoking habit. Some pharmacists might question the person about how many cigarettes are smoked, when they are smoked, and so on. However, where time is of the essence, and this is often the case, it can be argued that such questioning is not necessary, since the most important factor is that the person has made the decision to stop and this should be supported by the pharmacist. It may be useful to ask if the person has tried to stop before and, if so, whether they have taken any products at that time.

Since this person has directly asked about anti-smoking products it then becomes the pharmacist's professional decision whether or not to recommend the sale of such a product. While the pharmacist knows that it is unlikely to be the pharmacological action of the product which helps the customer to stop, the customer might welcome the psychological support of a product. However, the pharmacist must point out that there is no 'magic cure' for stopping smoking.

The pharmacist can explain the Health Education Authority guidelines, as we have mentioned previously, and can link this to 'Stop Smoking' leaflets which are available from the local Health Promotion Unit or direct from the Health Education Authority. It is important, in encouraging the person to read the leaflet later, to connect the advice given to what is written in the leaflet.

The pharmacist can suggest that the customer comes back to the pharmacy to report progress. Common sequelae of stopping smoking include the worsening of an existing cough as the cilia in the lungs begin to beat again (their action is stopped by smoking) and also irritability and nervous tension. The pharmacist can explain that these effects are likely to occur and that they will normally pass within a week or two. The key points are as follows:

- To welcome the decision to stop;

- To give structured advice;

- To support the advice by written information and to invite return to the pharmacy to report progress.

'Oh, I'm going to stop smoking on "No Smoking Day"—the trouble is, I've always put on lots of weight when I've tried before.'

A woman aged about thirty is discussing the subject of smoking with the pharmacist after noticing the supply of leaflets about 'National No Smoking Day'. For some people who stop smoking, the habit of eating can replace the habit of smoking. Comfort foods which are high in fat may well be consumed, leading to an increase in weight. There is no doubt that, in terms of the health risk of coronary heart disease, smoking is far more dangerous than being overweight. However, for many customers, especially women, smoking may seem to be the lesser of the two evils. Since the metabolic rate is increased by nicotine in cigarette smoke, stopping smoking may have the initial effect that weight will be gained. Exercise can help to raise the metabolic rate and the diet should be low in fat and sugar and high in fibre. The customer could chew sugar-free gum as a substitute habit. The pharmacist may also give advice and information on healthy eating generally. Putting on weight after stopping smoking is not inevitable and the pharmacist can give dietary advice about how to avoid weight gain if this is likely to be a problem.

'What have you got for a cough?'

A middle-aged man who works as a labourer at the local foundry is a regular visitor to the pharmacy in the winter months for cough mixtures. The pharmacist's normal questioning series, *WHAM*—

*W*ho is the medicine for and what are the symptoms?, *H*ow long have they been present?, *A*ny action taken (particularly medicines tried already)?, and what regular *M*edication is already being taken)?'—is unlikely to reveal whether or not a person is a smoker unless the direct question is asked. Since about one-third of the population smoke, it would not be unreasonable for the pharmacist to ask a customer complaining of a cough this question, although it will be difficult to achieve this in a tactful way.

This is a situation where the pharmacist could offer opportunistic health education advice to a smoker. In addition to recommending the over-the-counter remedy that the customer has come in to buy, the pharmacist may gently ask any question, such as: 'Have you ever thought about stopping smoking?'. Market research has shown that two-thirds of smokers say they would like to give up.

Depending on the response, the pharmacist might then offer a leaflet about stopping smoking. When the health behaviour has reached the point of producing chronic symptoms—in this case, coughing—the person is more likely to be receptive to advice on changing that behaviour. The pharmacist might discuss how to stop smoking, offer to include a leaflet in the bag with the cough medicine, and invite the person to return to the pharmacy. In taking opportunities to discuss health promotion in the context of patients' symptoms the pharmacist must accept that sometimes her or his enquiries and advice will be rebuffed. However, a tactful and sympathetic approach might sometimes produce a positive response.

8 Alcohol

Alcohol misuse is a major health and social problem in today's society. The objective for alcohol, in contrast to tobacco, is not to prevent people from starting to drink but to reduce average levels of drinking throughout the community. In their everyday practice pharmacists in hospital and community are commonly asked whether alcohol can be drunk while taking a particular medicine. Direct requests for advice about the effects of alcohol on health are fewer, but the pharmacist may be asked for reassurance or advice about, for example, a spouse's drinking levels. The pharmacist, therefore, needs to understand safe drinking limits for men and women, the extent of alcohol use in our society, and the medical and social problems which result.

8.1 Definitions of problem drinking

In their 1987 report, *The medical consequences of alcohol abuse*, the Royal College of Physicians attempted to define different levels of problem drinking and these are shown below. However, all such classifications are arbitrary, and terms such as 'alcoholic', although widely used in our society, are impossible to define.

Definitions of different kinds of drinkers

1. *Social drinker*. Someone who drinks usually not more than 2–3 units of alcohol a day and does not become intoxicated, is not likely to harm him- or herself or family through drinking. The amount that can be drunk without harm varies widely between individuals, but greater amounts than this are associated with increasing risk of harm.

2. *Heavy drinker*. Someone who regularly drinks more than 6 units of alcohol a day but without apparent immediate harm.

3. *Problem drinker*. Someone who experiences physical,

psychological, social, family, occupational, financial, or legal problems attributable to drinking.

4. *Dependent drinker.* Someone who has a compulsion to drink; takes roughly the same amount each day; has increased tolerance to alcohol in the early stages and reduced tolerance later; suffers withdrawal symptoms if alcohol is stopped which are relieved by consuming more; in whom drinking takes precedence over other activities and who tends to resume drinking after a period of abstinence.

Estimates of the numbers of people at risk from problem drinking were made by the Office of Health Economics in 1981 and are shown in Table 8.1, below.

These definitions and estimates show clearly that the alcohol problem is not, contrary to popular opinion, confined to 'alcoholics', but to a far higher proportion of the population. Market research has shown that the public are well informed of the dangers of 'alcoholism' but that there is little awareness of the widespread medical and social damage by lower levels of drinking which are nevertheless harmful to health and becoming endemic. It is in this area of the dissemination of information as to what constitutes safe levels of drinking, the hazards that result from over-indulgence in alcohol, and the alternatives available, that the community pharmacist has—as do all other members of the primary healthcare team— a role to play.

Table 8.1 Types of problem drinker and numbers at risk

Type	Estimate of number at risk in England and Wales	Per cent of population
Heavy drinking (showing biochemical abnormality)	3 million	8
Problem drinking (drinking which results in harm to the drinker or others)	700 000	2
Alcohol dependence	150 000	0.4

(Source: 'Alcohol: reducing the harm', Office of Health Economics 1981)

8.2 Epidemiology

8.2.1 Morbidity and mortality

Alcohol-associated deaths due to cirrhosis, accidents, suicide, and other causes are greatly underestimated, partly because doctors signing death certificates may be reluctant to identify alcohol as a cause because to do so would invoke the stigma of alcohol misuse and increase the family's grief. Another major reason for under-reporting is lack of awareness of the part played by alcohol in causing an individual's death. The Royal College of Physicians in their 1987 report *The medical consequences of alcohol abuse* estimated that alcohol is responsible for 25 000 premature deaths each year in men aged 35–64. Alcohol-associated morbidity is even more difficult to determine; the Office of Health Economics has estimated that 8–15 million working days are lost each year because of alcohol-related illness.

Excess alcohol consumption leads to both physical and mental ill-health. One in five of all acute male hospital admissions to medical wards in the UK are associated with alcohol and one-third of patients attending casualty departments have a blood alcohol concentration above 80 mg/100 ml (the legal limit for driving purposes). It is thought that many elderly people who are admitted to hospital because of falls, confusion, heart failure, and recurrent chest infections, may have alcohol problems. There were almost 18 000 alcohol-related admissions to mental hospitals in England and Wales in 1981.

8.2.2 Family problems and domestic violence

It is not only the drinkers themselves who suffer—their wives and families often suffer mental and physical abuse. Alcohol problems are frequently cited as a contributor to marital problems and divorce. Alcohol misuse undoubtedly contributes to domestic violence. In one British study, over half of the battered wives interviewed described their husbands as 'frequently drunk' and a further one-fifth said there were 'episodes of heavy drinking with drunkenness'.

8.2.3 Alcohol and driving

Road traffic accidents and the resultant morbidity and mortality are alcohol-related in many cases. The 1967 Road Safety Act introduced the Breathalyser and made it illegal to drive a motor vehicle with a blood alcohol level of over 80 mg/100 ml. However, convictions for drunken driving rose in the mid-1970s and by 1980 they were ten times the 1967 level in England and Wales. There were 85 000 convictions for drunken driving in 1983.

8.2.4 Problems at work and unemployment

Although most problem drinkers are still in employment, they have an increased likelihood of accidents and a significantly higher level of absenteeism. A major Swedish study showed that those men whose serum gamma-glutyl-transpeptidase (GGT) levels were in the top 10 per cent of the population had some 60 days' sick leave each year, five times as many as those below the median. In addition to accidents and ill-health, judgement and decision-making are likely to be impaired in problem drinkers, and the costs of this area of alcohol-related problems are impossible to calculate.

Many studies have looked at the alcohol consumption of unemployed people, with confusing and contradictory results. Possible reasons for the difficulty in discerning consistent patterns are that excess alcohol consumption may come before and even precipitate unemployment, that the poverty associated with unemployment influences alcohol purchases, and that the definition of employment influences the groups studied. For example, one study showed a drop in the alcohol consumption of unemployed men but a substantial rise in alcohol consumption among retired men.

The estimated social cost of alcohol misuse in England and Wales in 1985 is illustrated in Table 8.2.

Problem drinking occurs across all social groups, although some studies have shown that men in manual occupations drink more than those in non-manual occupations, while others have shown no relationship between alcohol consumption and social class. The relationship between social classification and alcohol consumption is not clear-cut and is interrelated with income level. Young people tend to drink more than those in older age groups and young single working men in their early- to mid-20s are the heaviest drinkers.

Table 8.2   The social cost of alcohol misuse—England and Wales, 1985

Consequence	Cost
To industry (loss of productivity and unemployment)	£1600 millions
To the NHS (hospital and community)	£104 millions
To society in its response (health education and research)	£1 million
In material damage and criminal activities (police and court costs)	£142 millions
In domestic disharmony and suffering	£1847 millions

There is growing evidence that alcohol misuse may be increasing among women. Young people are likely to drink regularly before the age of 18 (a major survey showed that under-age drinking is common in 65 per cent of 16–17-year-olds).

Unlike smoking cigarettes, drinking alcohol is not always harmful to health. Indeed, it is part of our cultural heritage—the pub is still very much a centre of social activity in the UK, and special occasions such as weddings and family reunions are normally accompanied by drinking alcohol in one form or another. This is also recognized in commonly expressed sentiments—'The cup that cheers', 'A little wine for thy stomach's sake'—and the great majority (over 90 per cent) of the adult population drink alcohol to some extent.

During the first half of this century there was a fall in beer consumption, which began with the First World War. Consumption rose sharply during the Second World War, fell during the post-war period, but rose again from 1960 onwards. Britain is traditionally a beer-drinking country and beer still represents 60 per cent of the total alcohol market. But wine consumption has more than quadrupled and spirits consumption doubled since 1960, while beer consumption fell by 15 per cent between 1979 and 1985.

Some of the reasons for the increase in consumption seen since the 1950s include the wide availability of alcohol, with many sales outlets, including supermarkets as well as traditional off-licences and, in recent years, the popularity of home-brewed beer and wine. The number of outlets selling alcohol increased by 40 per cent from 1973, to 180 000 in 1983. Like tobacco, the consumption of alcohol is price-sensitive, so that price is an important determinant of consumption. In recent years the *real* price of alcohol has fallen. Between 1978 and 1985 the 'work equivalent' of a bottle of whisky fell from 2 hours 24 minutes to 2 hours 11 minutes and the percentage of disposable income spent on alcohol increased from 7.3 per cent to 7.4 per cent. Wide advertising of alcohol on television and in magazines and newspapers continues with large sums of money spent on its promotion.

8.3 Health risks from alcohol

The serious medical consequences of alcohol abuse are many and include cirrhosis of the liver, cerebrovascular disease, pancreatitis, brain damage, heart failure, hypertension, and oesophageal cancer, where high alcohol consumption significantly increases the cancer risk. Less dangerous but nevertheless disabling are the nausea and retching which accompany alcoholic gastritis.

Ingestion of alcohol by a pregnant woman can lead to permanent damage to the child, including abnormal growth and mental retardation. Moderate drinking (less than 10 units per week) at the time of conception or during pregnancy does not appear to pose any risk to the fetus. Research has shown that women are at greater physical risks than are men for equivalent amounts of alcohol.

Over one-third of fatal road accidents are alcohol-related, and one-fifth of admissions to psychiatric hospitals are associated with alcohol consumption higher than recommended limits. Domestic violence, strife, and child abuse are often alcohol-related, and assault and criminal damage are frequently the result of excess alcohol. Table 8.3 summarizes some of the major ways in which alcohol harms health.

To summarize, alcohol is widely advertised, readily accessible, and is, in real terms, cheaper than it has been in the recent past. This has resulted in widespread use of, and in over-indulgence in, alcohol, with many social and medical consequences.

8.4 Giving advice in the pharmacy

The pharmacist is well-placed to act as an informed health professional, giving the latest information and advice on safe drinking levels. The World Health Organization states that there is no such

Table 8.3 Alcohol misuse—some major indices of harm

Consequences of misuse	Degree of association with alcohol	Size of the problem in England and Wales, 1984
Cirrhosis of the liver	Risk proportional to daily consumption	2300 deaths
Cancers (mainly digestive)	3% of all cancers alcohol-related. 44-fold risk of oesophogeal cancer in smokers who drink heavily	Around 4000 deaths
Fatal road traffic accidents	35% alcohol-related	1500 deaths
High blood pressure	Risk increases with consumption	Unknown
Psycho-social alcohol-dependence	100%	17 000 admissions to psychiatric hospitals
Public drunkenness	100%	108 000 convictions
Drinking and driving	100%	85 000 convictions

(Source: *The nation's health—A strategy for the 1990s*, Smith, A., and Jacobson, B. 1988)

thing as a completely safe level of drinking, since there are so many variable factors. Examples of such factors include the number of years during which an individual has consumed alcohol and the growing evidence that women are less able to tolerate alcohol than are men, even allowing for differences in body weight.

However, recognizing that alcohol is part of our social and cultural background, the targets sought by the Health Education Authority by the year 2000 are to work towards a situation where men do not exceed 21 standard units of alcohol per week and women do not exceed 14 standard units. Hence, the behaviour change sought is to ensure that anyone who asks for advice is given the unambiguous message that to drink more than this amount of alcohol each week is harmful to health. There is no requirement, unlike in cigarette smoking, that every customer who seeks advice should be encouraged to give up completely. Apart from anything else, an unduly prohibitive approach is unlikely to achieve success.

On those occasions when a patient seeks advice about problem drinking, the pharmacist can offer information and refer the patient to a local agency for further advice and counselling.

In a community-pharmacy-based health education campaign conducted in the West Midlands in 1985 the following important points emerged:

1. Unlike health promotion material on other subjects, it was important that the leaflets relating to alcohol were in a leaflet stand which included other information. Thus, it was not obvious to other customers or staff when alcohol-related leaflets were being taken. In a controlled trial it was shown that many more leaflets were taken when 'disguised in a forest' in this way.

2. The pharmacist should be well-informed on local self-help groups and centres which can give advice to people who are concerned about their own or other family members' drinking habits. Of these, the local branches of Alcoholics Anonymous, Aquarius, and Alcohol Advice Centres should be identified. In the study mentioned above, pharmacists found it useful to have these names typed on a separate sheet of paper, to be handed to customers on request.

3. The pharmacist should also clearly understand what constitutes a unit of alcohol and be able to explain the equivalents—for example, that a glass of wine, a half pint of beer, a glass of sherry, and a single measure of whisky all provide one unit of alcohol.

4. In the pharmacy-based alcohol campaign, unlike other health education campaigns, very few people asked for direct counselling advice in the pharmacy. This is perhaps not surprising for such a sensitive subject, but there were still occasions on which people sought confirmation of their fears that their own or a family member's drinking was of an inappropriately high level.

5. Pharmacists found they needed to be on their guard not to give reassurance in response to off-the-cuff, 'joking' comments and questions which in fact sought reassurance that the customer's drinking levels were not unreasonably high.

Many pharmacists volunteered concerns about the blunt 'avoid alcohol' statement which accompanies many medicines. Some of their customers had openly admitted that they sometimes ignored this advice, and pharmacists found that they needed to be well-briefed and prepared to be flexible in agreeing when alcohol was absolutely prohibited or when it was simply a wise precaution, and the approach could be occasionally more flexible if the customer was, for example, going to have a glass of wine and remain at home for the rest of the evening. In other words, pharmacists had to be aware of the risk/benefit each time a medicine bearing an additional labelling statement about alcohol was issued.

8.5 What can the pharmacist do?

Arguably, the most important thing the pharmacist can do is, if his is one of the dwindling number of pharmacy premises which still has

---

The community pharmacist is well-placed to:

- understand the health risks of alcohol to the drinker, his family, and society;

- publicize the dangers of alcohol and the importance of staying within 'safe' limits;

- know the addresses of local centres which can give counselling support to drinkers and to their families;

- listen to problems in an uncensorious and non-judgmental manner;

- recognize when he or she may be being asked to give reassurance about drinking levels which are higher than safe limits and where such reassurance would be inappropriate (see Appendix 1, p. 196);

- explain the difference between different types of alcohol and units of measurement;

- be well-informed on the interaction between alcohol and medicines.

an alcohol licence, to consider very seriously whether selling alcohol is compatible with a role as a health-promoter. Various reasons are given by pharmacists who continue to sell alcohol—'Mine are the only licensed premises in the village', 'Well, older people have come to expect to buy their alcohol here' or 'I do very little business, it's simply a tradition'—but these appear spurious in the light of the serious hazards of alcohol misuse. The Council of the Royal Pharmaceutical Society has issued a statement which effectively precludes the sale of tobacco products from pharmacies on the grounds of professional ethics. We believe that a similar statement should be issued regarding alcohol sales; indeed, moves are being made in this direction by the Society's Council.

Before offering advice on safe levels of drinking, the pharmacist should be well-informed about the health risks of alcohol misuse. Good publicity and information material is available about alcohol and 'safe' levels of drinking. This should normally be obtainable through the local Health Promotion Unit, who should be able to help with supplies of a range of appropriate leaflets. Other associations, such as Alcohol Concern, have excellent posters and leaflets, but these would normally have to be purchased.

9   Nutrition

From the 1930s onwards, thinking and education on nutrition was based on the premise that the population should receive a balanced diet—that is, to prevent malnourishment. This was of great importance at a time of widespread economic deprivation and ensured that the population received sufficient amounts of protein, carbohydrate, minerals, and essential fats. A commonly-held belief developed that some foods were essentially 'good' (such as cheese) and others were inherently 'bad' (and in this category, all carbohydrates were grouped together, including bread and potatoes). Two major factors began to change this view in the 1970s—the rising death toll from coronary heart disease and the awareness that this was related to nutrition, and the rising percentage of processed food in the diet. Research evidence now shows that diet is linked to many diseases and symptoms. Coronary heart disease should be a major focus for dietary advice from the pharmacist because of its high incidence. Pharmacists are also in a good position to offer dietary advice about many other conditions.

9.1 Diet and disease

Research evidence gathered over the last three decades has gradually elucidated the interrelationship between diet and ill-health.

The link between diet and disease

- Cardiovascular conditions Coronary heart disease
  Hypertension
  Stroke

- Gastrointestinal tract Indigestion
  Heartburn
  Constipation
  Irritable bowel syndrome
  Diverticulosis
  Bowel cancer

- Allergy   Coeliac disease
                                   Lactose intolerance
                                   Eczema
                                   Hayfever
                                   Migraine
- Others   Vitamin deficiencies
                                   Eating disorders (anorexia,
                                   bulimia)

Mounting concern about diet and health led to the publication of two reports in the early 1980s which summarized current research evidence on nutrition and disease. The NACNE (National Advisory Committee on Nutrition Education) report, 1983, examined the diet of the British population in relation to a wide range of conditions and the COMA (The Committee on Medical Aspects of Food Policy) report, *Diet and cardiovascular disease*, 1984, specifically looked at diet and cardiovascular disease. Both were in broad agreement that the amount of total energy derived from dietary fat should be reduced, that there should be a reduction in the intake of saturated fat, and that there was some evidence to support a small increase in the intake of polyunsaturated fats. In 1988 the World Health Organization (WHO) published a report with recommendations for healthy eating in Europe, *Nutrition and health*, which proposed reductions in fats, sugar, and salt and an increase in dietary fibre. COMA published its report *Dietary sugars and human disease* in 1989.

The NACNE and WHO reports made some recommendations which were more specific than those in the COMA *Diet and cardiovascular disease* report. These were that the amount of sugar in the diet should be reduced, that less salt should be eaten, and that the amount of fibre in the diet should be increased. The NACNE report noted with concern the rise in consumption of dairy foods during the previous 15 years and that sugar was added to many foods but that the consumer had little idea of the sugar content.

Fibre is removed from many foods during processing and there is widespread public belief that all carbohydrates (and fibre is contained in many starchy carbohydrates such as pulses) were likely to cause an increase in weight. In the public's mind, therefore, carbohydrates were 'fattening' and should be avoided. In fact, excess calories and consequent weight gain were more likely to be because

of the amounts of saturated fats and sugar which were being consumed or the way in which carbohydrate foods, such as potatoes,
were being cooked—the British diet of 'chips with everything'.

The main dietary recommendations of these reports were as
follows:

1. *Fat intake*. The NACNE report recommended that the percentage of total energy derived from fat should be reduced from the
then current 42.6 per cent to 30 per cent. The report said that much
of this reduction could be achieved by eating fewer dairy foods—for
example, by moving from full fat to semi-skimmed milk, by eating
polyunsaturated spreads, and by reducing the amount of hard
cheese consumed. Reducing the amount of red meat and changing
to white meat such as chicken was another important means of
achieving this goal. Changing the method of cooking from frying to
grilling or baking, using vegetable oils if frying, effectively reduces
fat intake. The percentage recommended in the COMA *Diet and
cardiovascular disease* report was 35 per cent; the World Health
Organization's *Nutrition and health* recommendation was 30 per
cent. Simple changes could achieve this reduction—for example,
changing from full-fat to semi-skimmed milk would go almost
halfway to meeting the guidelines.

2. *Sugar*. The NACNE report recommended that the amount of
sugar consumed should decrease from the then current 38 kg per
head per annum to 20 kg. The recent COMA report *Dietary sugars
and human disease* makes no specific recommendation about reducing sugar intake but suggests that those people who consume
more than 200 g daily should replace the excess with starch. The
NACNE committee felt that much of its recommended reduction
could be achieved by better labelling and improved consumer
awareness of the sugar content of many foods. Most consumers
would expect that 'sweets' should contain sugar but be surprised to
learn that approximately four teaspoonsful of sugar are included in
a carton of standard fruit yoghurt and that sugar is contained in
powdered soups, baked beans, and products such as muesli. Sugar-
free and reduced sugar products are now on sale but many others
still contain large quantities of sugar.

3. *Salt*. The NACNE report recommended that the amount of
salt should be reduced by 3 g per day. The report recognized that

much of the salt we eat is hidden in processed food but obvious steps are to discontinue the habit of routinely adding salt when cooking and, instead, making it available at the table. Better consumer awareness is needed of the large quantity of salt contained in some foods such as yeast extracts and powdered soups. Food labelling should clearly state salt content.

4. *Fibre.* The NACNE report recommended that the amount of fibre we eat should rise from 20 g per day to 30 g. Most of this increase can be achieved by eating wholemeal bread (and there has already been a large switch in this direction), more potatoes (particularly unpeeled and cooked in any way other than fried), pulses, and root vegetables. There is a widespread, and misconceived, belief that to eat more fibre necessarily requires a diet high in salad vegetables, which are perceived as being very expensive. In fact, most salad vegetables contain very little fibre.

9.2 Health risks

9.2.1 The case for reducing fat in the diet

The major health risk is of coronary heart disease. The higher the cholesterol level in the blood, the greater the risk of heart disease. This risk is proportional to the extent to which the cholesterol level is raised (the 20 per cent of people with the nation's highest cholesterol levels are three times more likely to die of heart disease than the 20 per cent with the lowest levels). When blood cholesterol levels are reduced, either by drugs or diet, there is an equivalent reduction in the risk of heart disease. High cholesterol levels have been shown in major studies to be one of the three major modifiable risk factors for coronary heart disease (the other two being smoking and hypertension).

A diet which is high in fat is also likely to be high in calories and lead to weight gain. Thus, dietary fats contribute to the development of overweight and obesity, a further risk factor for heart disease.

The percentage of cholesterol in the blood which is derived from the cholesterol in our diet (from high-cholesterol foods such as egg yolk) is low. Cholesterol is produced by the liver in direct proportion to the amount of saturated fat that is eaten. A common misunderstanding among the public is that only foods which are high in cholesterol are 'bad'. Current thinking is that a cholesterol level of 5.2 mmol/litre or less is associated with a low risk of heart disease in people over 30 and 4.7 mmol/litre in people under 30 years. For the British population, recent studies suggest that over 60 per cent are therefore at risk—that is, they have levels above 5.2 mmol/litre. However, there is a strong case for changing the eating habits of the whole population to more healthy patterns, rather than concentrating simply on those individuals who have high cholesterol levels. Cholesterol measurement in the pharmacy can provide a powerful focus for dietary advice from the pharmacist.

Bowel cancer appears to be linked to a diet which is high in fat and red meat and low in fibre. Research has been unable to identify the contribution of the two factors, fat and fibre, to the development of bowel cancer. It is true that diets which are low in fibre are often high in fat and thus increasing fibre and reducing fats may protect against bowel cancer. The role of diet in bowel cancer is further discussed in Chapter 6, on p. 98.

There is also some evidence to link diets which are high in fat to certain cancers, notably those of breast and prostate.

9.2.2 The case for reducing salt

Salt intake appears to be one of the factors which affect blood pressure, and high blood pressure is a major contributory factor to heart disease and stroke. The incidence of stroke has been reduced over the last 10 years, largely due to the intervention of screening for hypertension and subsequent action either by drug therapy or changes such as weight reduction and reduced salt intake. While the WHO, NACNE, and COMA reports were agreed that salt intake in the UK is too high and that salt appears to play an important part in the development of hypertension, the evidence is not clear-cut.

Research has clearly shown that, in societies where salt intake is low, blood pressure does not rise with age, as is the case in the developed world. In those societies, the incidence of coronary heart disease and stroke are significantly lower. However, it has yet to be proved that a reduction in salt intake in individual diets in the UK has resulted in a proportional reduction in the incidence of hypertension. Population studies are fraught with difficulties—they must be longitudinal (that is, conducted over many years), take into account other changes in diet and lifestyle, and then demonstrate that one factor has affected the whole. Nonetheless, expert opinion is agreed that a reduction in salt in the diet is likely to be of benefit even though the case for it is not fully proven.

9.2.3 The case for reducing sugar

The most recent survey in the UK showed 45 per cent of males and 36 per cent of females to be overweight, with one in twelve men and one in eight women classified as obese (for definitions of these terms, see Chapter 4, p. 72). The percentage of the population who are obese has been increasing in the UK over a period of several decades. The process begins early in life; by the age of 11 years, 6 per cent of boys and 10 per cent of girls are overweight.

The major dietary contributory factors to weight gain are fats and sugar. At the time the NACNE report was published, the average sugar consumption in the UK was 38 kg per person annually— double the recommended level. Nutritionists are agreed that sugar is not an essential component of our diet; in fact sugar has been said to provide 'empty calories', that is, it has no nutritional value. There is increasing awareness that non-insulin-dependent diabetes is associated with obesity, although no direct causal role for excess sugar intake has been established.

Sugar is implicated in the onset of dental caries. The concern is that young children are most seriously at risk from dental caries, and it is they who are most likely to receive the heavily sugared products such as fizzy drinks and sweets which are liable to cause their teeth to rot. Criticism has been levelled at food manufacturers for not clearly stating sugar content, particularly in foods and drinks for babies.

9.2.4 The case for more fibre

All the major reports on nutrition have recommended an increase in dietary fibre as one of the measures to be taken in reducing the likelihood of coronary heart disease. In this case, the amount of fibre consumed affects the cholesterol level. Recent research suggests that this is due at least in part to an indirect effect—due to a reduction in the amount of saturated fats consumed when an individual increases the amount of fibre eaten. However, soluble fibre (found in oats, fruit, vegetables, and pulses) appears to have the effect of reducing cholesterol levels.

The second cause of concern as a result of our low-fibre diet is the incidence of bowel cancer, which is low in countries where fibre intake is high. While there is no definitive case that a low-fibre diet causes bowel cancer, and the picture is unclear because of the fact that low-fibre diets also tend to be high in fats, the Royal College of Physicians' report, *Medical aspects of dietary fibre*, considered this to be an important aspect as well as in other cancers and non-cancerous conditions.

The beneficial effect of increased fibre intake on the incidence of constipation is well-established. Constipation can range from being merely a troublesome symptom to having much more serious implications—such as the retention of potential toxins and car-cinogens in the dietary tract for days rather than hours (thought to increase cancer risk) and the likelihood of developing related con-ditions, such as diverticular disease or haemorrhoids (see also p. 143).

Other conditions which are linked to a low dietary fibre intake are diverticulosis and the irritable bowel syndrome. Patients suffering from either are likely to benefit from increasing their intake of fibre.

9.3 Dietary advice from the pharmacist

Eating is, for most people, doing far more than simply keeping malnutrition at bay. This is true even in primitive societies, where the tribe will gather together to share a meal. Food is associated with early childhood memories and pleasures, and what was offered as a treat in childhood is likely to remain so throughout life—witness expensive London restaurants offering food such as bread-and-butter pudding and steamed treacle sponge, remembered pre-sumably from happy schooldays and still much sought-after by middle-aged men.

So it is important to realize that many people cannot change their eating habits easily—if this were not the case, the population would not have such a high percentage of overweight men and women. The behaviour change sought, therefore, which is most likely to succeed, is not to eschew favoured foods totally but to 'ration' them and to substitute others which may become desired in their own right. Thus, if either chips—or, say, cream cakes—are seen to be desirable foods that the customer cannot live without, then it is pointless to suggest that they be abandoned but, rather, that they should be eaten for 'treats' on special occasions.

Alcoholic drinks contain a significant number of calories and, when reviewing the diet, consideration should be given to alcohol intake.

The following tables (9.1–9.4) show the foods that have the greatest percentage of fat, sugar and salt, and the lowest percentage of fibre, together with the substitutes that can most acceptably be offered.

9.4 Over-the-counter and prescription products

9.4.1 For weight loss

Pharmacists are regularly asked to advise about the best product for losing weight quickly, and 'slimming' products are also widely available from other outlets. What is the best advice? The micro diets are also known as VLCD (very low calorie diets) and have an intake of 600 calories per day or less. Many such products are in the form of a soup or sweet drink mixture, based on skimmed milk, with added vitamins and other nutrients. Such products will, because of their low calorific intake, lead to weight loss, but there are several concerns about their use.

For the people who are overweight (body mass index above 25— for definition, see Chapter 4, p. 72), and where there is no underlying health disorder, short-term use of a VLCD of up to four weeks should pose no risk. However, the long-term effects of a continued calorie intake which is very low are less clear and the loss of lean tissue in addition to fat can lead to problems. VLCDs have received much publicity, and therefore close attention, since in the past they have been the occasion of fatalities. In each case, the women had adhered rigidly to the diet for far longer than the manufacturer's

Table 9.1 Fat content of foods

High	*Low*
All fried food, sausages, pate, dairy foods (butter, cream, hard cheeses, full-fat milk), red meat (except lean cuts), mayonnaise, salad cream, suet, potato crisps, meat pies and pasties, margarine	Semi-skimmed and skimmed milk, cottage cheese, low fat yoghurt, Grilled fish, white meat (turkey, chicken, rabbit), all vegetables, potatoes (other than fried), cereals, low fat cheese, low fat spreads

Table 9.2 Foods with a high sugar content

Food	Sugar content
Soft drinks	4–8 teaspoonfuls per glass
Desserts	
Ice Cream (family block)	9 teaspoonfuls of sugar
Jelly (one packet)	19 teaspoonfuls of sugar
Fruit yoghurt (one carton)	4 teaspoonfuls of sugar
Tinned fruit (one small tin)	5 teaspoonfuls of sugar
Cereals, (where sugar is included)	1–2 teaspoonsful per serving
Biscuits	one biscuit =1 to 2 teaspoonfuls of sugar
Cakes	one slice = 1 to 4 teaspoonfuls of sugar
Sweet sauces, custard	one serving = 1 teaspoonful of sugar
Soups (tinned/packet)	one bowl = 1–2 teaspoonfuls of sugar
Tinned vegetables	small tin = 1 to 2 teaspoonfuls of sugar
Confectionery	All confectionery is likely to comprise over 50% sugar.

recommendation and the muscle loss was sufficiently great to weaken vital heart muscle. Those products currently available have been reformulated and manufacturers' instructions refer to short periods of use. Some people should not use VLCDs at all—these include pregnant women, diabetics, those with heart disease, and children.

However, the major drawback of very low calorie diets is that healthier eating patterns are not learned. When the diet is stopped research shows that the majority of people regain their lost weight and even increase from their starting weight.

Thus, while pharmacists may continue to stock and sell these products on their judgment, the very clear added instruction should be given that they should not be taken for more than four weeks and only after having ensured that it is safe for that particular customer to do so. At the same time, advice can be offered on the way of achieving weight loss that is likely to be maintained. An agreed change in diet between the pharmacist and the customer is more

Table 9.3   High-salt foods

Salted peanuts, peanut butter, crisps, yeast extracts

Hard cheeses, bacon, processed meat, sausages, pork/beef pies, smoked
   fish

Some breakfast cereals (All Bran, cornflakes), tinned and packet soups,
   tinned and packet vegetables

---

likely to have long-term results. One helpful measure is to ask the
customer to keep a diary of everything they eat during the course of
a week. It is then easy to identify the parts of the diet which are
likely to be causing an increase in weight for reasons of which the
customer may be unaware. Group support has been shown to be an
effective way of maintaining weight loss, and the Weight Watchers
organization is one of the few slimming aids found to be effective by
the Consumers' Association. Referral to a dietitian for further
advice and counselling is another option and pharmacists can
contact their local dietitians to establish working links.

Other proprietary products sold to help those wishing to lose
weight are designed as meal substitutes of known and low calorie
content, or to prevent hunger pangs by their fibre content. Good
advice from the pharmacist about high-fibre foods which can
achieve the same effect can be helpful. The fibre content of many
slimming products such as bran tablets is relatively low, and increasing dietary fibre in other ways is a healthier alternative. The
'natural' snack bars containing dried fruit, bran, and oats are often
high in sugar and are not a low-calorie alternative to sweets.
Labelling information on such products states the sugar content.

Artificial sweeteners such as 'Nutrasweet' have largely replaced
traditional saccharin which had the disadvantage of an unpleasantly
bitter after-taste. In addition to sweetening tablets for hot drinks,

Table 9.4   Fibre content of foods

High	Low
Pulses—peas, lentils, etc., wholemeal bread, dried fruit, baked beans, bananas, oranges, brown rice, wholewheat pasta, potatoes in their skins, root vegetables, most leaf vegetables, nuts	Lettuce, cucumber, tomato, white bread, white rice, white pasta

granulated forms are now available which taste virtually the same as sugar. Soft drinks and dessert products are only two of a wide range of artificially-sweetened foods. While the ideal is to reduce or cut out sugar completely, such products can be helpful for those who find it difficult to give up sweet-tasting foods from their diet.

9.4.2 Laxatives

Many pharmacy customers ask for treatment for constipation and, since the most common cause of constipation is insufficient fibre and fluids in the diet, advice on cheap and effective ways of dealing with this are likely to give long-term benefits. Once the pharmacist has identified from questioning that the constipation is due to dietary causes, advice can be given about ways in which to increase fibre intake. However, it is nearly always the case that customers seeking a laxative from the pharmacist are likely to need relief from their uncomfortable symptoms quickly. There is no reason why the pharmacist should not recommend a laxative for short-term use to relieve the immediate problem. High-fibre foods are better introduced gradually into the diet, and increasing dietary fibre will take up to a week to improve gut motility and stool consistency. If the person needs quicker relief, one or two doses of a stimulant laxative such as bisacodyl or senna can be supplied which will produce a bowel motion within twelve hours. The key point here is to supply the minimum quantity needed and to explain that the laxative will deal with the current discomfort but that dietary change is essential. Bulk laxatives such as ispaghula and sterculia will take two to three days to produce a bowel motion and are an alternative where immediate relief from symptoms is not required.

Haemorrhoids (piles) are often caused by the straining which accompanies constipation, and the guidelines given above can be used to offer advice about reducing discomfort from haemorrhoidal symptoms associated with constipation and preventing their recurrence.

While it is outside the scope of this book to discuss the differentiation of symptom causation, it is important to emphasize that prolonged change in bowel habit in anyone aged over 50, particularly if accompanied by rectal bleeding, requires immediate medical referral. Bowel cancer is rare in those aged under 50 and commonly presents as a sustained change in bowel habit (particularly constipation).

There is widespread misunderstanding among the public as to which foods are high in fibre. Leaflets or other written information about the fibre content of specific foods can be most helpful. Encouraging customers to read food labels while shopping can also be helpful in identifying good sources of fibre. The Health Education Authority produces a range of leaflets on nutrition, which can be stocked by the pharmacist.

9.5 Case studies

The opportunities for advice on healthy eating are interwoven everywhere into pharmacy practice. From the customer who complains of heartburn after meals to those complaining of constipation and haemorrhoids, there are opportunities everywhere for the pharmacist to offer good advice. To do so, pharmacists need to be informed on the key risk areas and also to recognize the important part that diet plays in the whole lifestyle. Women form the majority of pharmacy customers and it is largely they who determine what food will be bought for the family. But they must always strike a balance between good advice which may be given by the pharmacist and what their families will actually eat, ranging from pernickety children to husbands who are set in their dietary ways. Thus, the pharmacist will need to listen with care to what the customer says about the family's likes before deciding on key areas where change could be effected.

'My husband's just come out of the hospital. We've had such a fright—he had a heart attack. He's on tablets for his high blood pressure now but he's been told to cut down on fats and to lose some weight. He's 12 stones and should be 11 stones. Have you got any good diet sheets?'

'My husband's had his cholesterol done at the doctor's—it was over 7. How can he get it down? And should I change my diet as well?'

Here the key issue is to reduce saturated fat, and in the first case also to reduce salt. Care should be taken in giving this advice that customers are put onto a weight-reduction diet only where needed, based on their body mass index. Where weight loss is not necessary, the amount of saturated fat should be reduced without calorie reduction by reducing the amount of dairy food and red meat, and poultry, fish, and carbohydrates (pulses, potatoes, and wholemeal bread) should be used as their replacement. Verbal advice should be supported by written material in the form of easily-understood leaflets. The Pharmaceutical Services Negotiating Committee produces a suitable leaflet for dietary advice in conjunction with cholesterol measurement. Ideally the pharmacist will be able to monitor blood pressure and cholesterol levels where appropriate. Referral to a dietitian might be considered, particularly where dietary change has not produced a reduction in cholesterol after 3–5 months.

'Well, here I am again. It's another April and I'm 2 stones overweight. I tried that micro diet last year and it really worked, so I suppose I'll try it again. What do you think?'

Advice needs to be given with sensitivity here as to what is an achievable goal, bearing in mind the amount of pleasure that may be derived from a plate of chips or a cream cake. Where the pharmacy has facilities for weighing and measuring height, the body mass index can be calculated and advice given accordingly. A person with a BMI of over 25 is generally considered to be 'overweight', and of over 30 'obese'. Weight reduction is best achieved by reduction in fat intake, particularly of saturated fat, and by reducing the amount of sugar that is eaten. The pharmacist should explain that starchy foods such as potatoes and pulses are filling and nutritious. Finally but very importantly, taking more exercise will help in the weight loss programme. The pharmacist can keep a stock of weight recording sheets and can invite the customer to return to the pharmacy to monitor progress. Referral to the dietitian could be considered if the appropriate weight loss is not achieved.

'But I can't afford it—these healthy foods are too expensive. And anyway I haven't got time.'

Some of the recommended advice on better eating habits may mean higher expenditure on food. Several studies have shown that the diet of people living on unemployment benefit is likely to consist of a high percentage of processed food, tinned food, white bread, and high-sugar foods. The reasons are very simple: they are the cheapest to buy, the energy required to heat and serve them is very low, and they can be purchased locally—very important considerations for people who cannot afford bus fares to a supermarket. Nonetheless, there is much advice that can be offered to show, for example, that high-fibre foods need not be expensive, including potatoes, wholemeal bread (although this is always more expensive than white), and baked beans. Fat can also be reduced in cost-efficient ways such as the use of polyunsaturated spreads and semi-skimmed milk. Care should be taken that high-cost suggestions are not made to those on reduced incomes, such as baking potatoes in their jackets when no other foods are to be cooked in the oven, since high energy use and cost will result. However, while the microwave oven continues to make its appearance in large numbers of households with a range of incomes, a cheap and rapid way to cook potatoes in their jackets may be available. For working mothers who want to prepare meals quickly, tinned pulses are a good source of fibre and an alternative to the lengthy soaking and cooking process of raw pulses. These few examples show the way in which advice can be fitted to the individual customer.

'What have you got for heartburn? I get it terribly after meals and when I go to bed.'

Heartburn and gastro-oesophageal reflux are symptoms where health education advice is more important than treatment with over-the-counter medicines. Being overweight is a major cause of heartburn, and advice on weight reduction can be given where appropriate. General healthy eating advice is relevant—eating meals with a lower fat content will help to reduce the symptoms of heartburn by decreasing the length of time for which food remains in the stomach. Reducing alcohol intake can be helpful, since alcohol makes the sphincter between the stomach and oesophagus less effective. Smoking has a similar effect and cutting down or stopping will lead to an improvement in the problem. While this, like alcohol consumption, can be a sensitive area to introduce into the conversation, the pharmacist can simply offer information in a non-judgemental way about the contribution which smoking and alcohol make to heartburn. Eating small meals often rather than the standard three meals each day means that the stomach is less full, and therefore its contents are less likely to leak back into the oesophagus. Finally, avoiding eating full meals within an hour or two of bedtime should help, and the pharmacist can supply a small quantity of antacid to help until the lifestyle measures begin to take effect.

10 Baby and child health

Mothers of young children are a major group of pharmacy customers and will ask the pharmacist about many aspects of baby and child health. Often such queries will relate to specific symptoms but in many cases it is general health advice and reassurance which is needed. In this sense the pharmacist, and to some extent the GP and health visitor, are being used as sources of advice and information because of the lack of advice from other family members: in the past, young mothers would often have obtained such advice from their own mothers based on experience. There is an important role for the pharmacist to give accurate, current and relevant advice in this area.

Baby and child health are subjects which are not usually included in undergraduate pharmacy courses. They are, however, areas in which it is vital for the pharmacist to be informed, to know when to refer to the doctor or clinic and when to allay fears. There are four main areas for advice:

1. practical aspects, e.g. infant feeding;

2. common and recurrent public health problems, e.g. head lice, threadworms;

3. topical issues, e.g. research on vitamins and intelligence;

4. common misconceptions, e.g. that antibiotics are always needed in infections.

Practical advice is often needed about routine aspects of caring for a baby, such as feeding choice and practice and for the treatment of common problems such as nappy rash, where the pharmacist can also offer advice about preventing recurrence. Awareness of current practice is essential where there has been a change in thinking—for example, about when to introduce cow's milk into the baby's diet.

Some problems are seasonal and regular—for example, an epidemic of head lice at the local school, when the pharmacist must know the district policy on choice of insecticide and be able to give advice on the use of products.

Others will be prompted by media publicity. A recurrent example of this is the sensational reports of brain damage caused by whooping cough vaccination, where what is needed from the pharmacist is an appraisal of the relative risks and benefits. For such issues of topical concern, the pharmacist is able to give the facts, where these are clearly known, or to make an appraisal of the evidence to date, and to err on the side of caution where there is any doubt.

The pharmacist has an important role in putting false hopes and fears into perspective—for example, expectations that vitamin supplementation will increase children's intelligence. Correcting widespread and deeply-held misconceptions is another important area for pharmacists' advice—for example, the idea that antibiotic therapy is always needed in the treatment of infections. Concerned parents may seek advice from the pharmacist about their child's prescription, and a clear explanation together with reassurance are needed.

We will now look at some key areas in baby and child health.

10.1 Vaccination and immunization

While vaccination may not generate many direct enquiries to the pharmacist, it is nevertheless essential that the pharmacist is aware of current vaccination schedules and knows the rationale behind each in order to respond should queries arise. With the increasing emphasis on preventive care and the requirement to reach certain targets in the new GP contract, parents are more likely to be contacted to ensure their children are vaccinated. Pharmacies would be a natural place to display leaflets on vaccination and these may generate questions in the informal atmosphere of the pharmacy. Indeed, the pharmacist may take a more pro-active role, offering such leaflets when dispensing prescriptions for babies and young children.

The current vaccination schedule is shown below.

Vaccination schedule for infants and children

1. In the first year of life, three doses of diphtheria, pertussis and polio vaccines. The first is given at two months of age, the second at three months and the third at four months.

2. In the second year of life, the measles, mumps, and rubella (MMR) vaccine is given, generally between 12–15 months.

3. At school entry, or entry to nursery school, diphtheria and polio vaccine boosters are given, and currently MMR vaccine is given until the children who received this vaccine in the second year of life reach school age.

4. Between the tenth and fourteenth birthdays, the BCG vaccine is given for tuberculin-negative children; girls are also given rubella vaccine between their tenth and fourteenth birthdays.

10.1.1 Pertussis (whooping cough)

Some 10 000 cases of pertussis were notified in 1989. Following many media reports of brain damage caused by pertussis vaccine, the percentage of infants who were vaccinated fell drastically during the 1970s. While the link between pertussis vaccine and brain damage is contentious and still provokes much debate, there is no doubt that the disease itself can cause brain damage. Estimates are that 1 in 500 cases of whooping cough result in brain damage, and the disease can be fatal. For the vaccine, epidemiological studies estimate that 1 in 100 000 injections resulted in a neurological reaction, most of which involved prolonged febrile convulsions from which most infants recovered without adverse consequences.

10.1.2 Measles, mumps, and rubella (MMR)

The measles, mumps, and rubella vaccine was introduced in October 1988 with the aim of eliminating congenital rubella syndrome, measles, and mumps. While many people consider rubella, measles, and mumps to be 'harmless' diseases of childhood, many problems result from their incidence. Measles has unpleasant complications, including encephalitis, which can be fatal. In adults mumps can cause orchitis (inflammation of the testes) in males and even sterility. Congenital rubella syndrome results where damage is done to the developing fetus when the mother becomes infected with rubella (German measles) during pregnancy. Multiple congenital defects—including heart problems, deafness, and cataracts—may occur.

After-effects following MMR include malaise, fever, and rash, usually about a week after the injection. Paracetamol syrup can be given and tepid spongeing to reduce the temperature. Parents should be reminded that spongeing with cold water can cause a further rise in temperature by shutting down blood vessels close to the skin surface, thereby reducing heat loss through the skin. Tepid water should, therefore, be used. Swelling of the parotid glands (those which are affected by mumps) can also occur, at a later stage of around three weeks after vaccination.

10.1.3 Contra-indications to vaccination

Contra-indications to vaccination is an area where there is much misunderstanding among both health professionals and members of the public. Vaccination should be postponed if the child is suffering from a febrile illness because the body's immune system is already activated and may destroy the vaccine before antibodies are made. Minor infections without fever or systemic upset are not contra-indications.

It is widely believed by members of the public and others that children who suffer from eczema or other allergic conditions should not receive vaccinations. This is emphatically *not* the case. Allergy to egg in the case of vaccines manufactured using chick embryos is only a contra-indication if the child has previously had an ana-phylactic reaction after eating eggs. Dislike of eggs or refusal to eat eggs is not a contra-indication.

The British National Formulary sets out advice on contra-indications for each vaccine and advises that the doctor should seek specialist advice from the local paediatrics department before deciding not to vaccinate a child.

10.1.4 Paracetamol in feverish reactions

Pharmacists may be asked if paracetamol can be given to infants aged under three months who become feverish following the first dose of diphtheria, pertussis, and polio vaccination. The British National Formulary recommends a dose of 5–10 mg/kg on the advice of a doctor. Guidelines are that for two month-old full-term infants 40 mg should be given and that for 2 month-old pre-term infants 10 mg/kg should be given. The small doses involved mean that oral syringes will be required to measure the dose.

10.2 Infant feeding

Most young mothers will seek advice from the health visitor or baby clinic about feeding and this advice will be of a high standard. Advice is also sought from pharmacists, and current thinking is that, while it is entirely appropriate for pharmacists to encourage breast-feeding and to give advice which will facilitate this, it is not the pharmacist's role to take positive steps to suggest that a baby is fed with a formula milk. Thus, if the mother is experiencing difficulties in breast-feeding, she should be referred to her health visitor, GP, or baby clinic to discuss the problems being encountered. If a formula feed is required, advice will then be given about its selection. Where a mother has been advised by the health visitor to use a formula feed or has decided independently to choose to bottle-feed rather than breast-feed, then it is appropriate for the pharmacist to offer advice about the selection of a product and its correct use.

10.2.1 Breast-feeding

Expert opinion is agreed that breast-feeding is best for all babies and confers several benefits. Research has shown clearly that breast-feeding, even if only for a period of 12 weeks, will give the baby protection against a variety of infections, particularly those of the respiratory tract. Almost all formula feeds are modified cows' milk and, whilst technical developments have meant that the nutritional composition of these milks has been made closely to resemble that of breast milk, the nature of the protein is different. Breast milk is the most easily digestible and is always preferable to formula milks.

Be mindful, when issuing prescription medicines or over-the-counter medicines for breast-feeding mothers, of the transfer of some drugs into the breast milk. The British National Formulary summarizes those drugs which are transferred in this way in its section on 'Prescribing during breast-feeding'. There has been publicity about the possible effects of coffee-drinking by breast-feeding mothers. Young babies are known to metabolize caffeine more slowly than adults and irritability in a baby whose mother consumes a lot of tea or coffee may be helped by a switch to decaffeinated versions. Fizzy drinks such as cola can be high in caffeine, so caffeine-free varieties are to be preferred.

Mothers may sometimes ask for advice about breast-feeding and the pharmacy should stock a range of the accessories and equipment to facilitate this. When the baby feeds at one breast, milk leaks from the other, and breast shells made of moulded plastic can be worn to collect the drips of milk. They should be sterilized before use. Breast pads are worn to catch drops of milk. They can be worn continuously to prevent wetting of clothes and are available in disposable and washable versions. A breast pump can be used to express milk which can then be stored in the fridge; the milk can also be frozen so long as it is used within four weeks. Nipple shields protect the skin and creams are available for sore or cracked nipples. If the nipples are very painful the mother should be advised to see her GP, as infection may have occurred.

10.2.2 Bottle-feeding

The range of baby milks on the pharmacy shelf can be very confusing and we will give a brief guide here to the different types. Whey-based milks (for example, Cow and Gate Premium, SMA Gold Cap) have formulae closest to breast milk and are most easily digested by the baby. Curd-based milks (for example, Cow and Gate Plus, SMA White Cap) contain a higher proportion of curd protein (casein) and are said to be more satisfying for hungrier babies, since the curds will stay in the stomach for longer and take longer to digest, giving a feeling of fullness. Other formula milks include those which are soya-based and suitable for babies who are allergic to cow's milk. Symptoms of such allergy include crying after feeds, vomiting, and diarrhoea. Fortunately, most babies 'grow out of' their allergy by the age of two years. Low-lactose feeds are designed to be given following a bout of gastroenteritis, when a temporary lactose intolerance is not uncommon. After the first six months of life, 'follow-on' milks are available (such as 'Progress') which are given until the end of the first year.

A good policy is to become familiar with one or two product ranges and to get up-to-date literature from the company representatives about new developments. Remember always to include a verbal reinforcement of the manufacturer's written advice about hygiene and sterilization of bottles and teats, and about the many infections that are transmitted via inadequately cleaned feeding equipment.

10.2.3 Cow's milk and babies

Cow's milk should never be introduced into the baby's diet before the age of one year. Because of the growing baby's need for calories, *semi-skimmed milk* (red/silver top) should not be given below the age of *two* years and *skimmed* (blue top) milk not below *five* years. Semi-skimmed and skimmed milks should only be given to children of the appropriate ages if their diet is satisfactory in terms of calorie and nutrient intake.

10.2.4 Crying and colic

Babies have been observed to cry characteristically and draw up their legs in the early evenings after feeds up to the age of three months. Such crying was thought to be due to colic ('three-month colic') and babies were given gripe water and other remedies. Research now suggests that the crying pattern has no connection with symptoms and that, while early-evening crying does reach a peak between the ages of two and three months, there was no evidence of symptoms in most babies. Some infants undoubtedly suffer from wind and here a silicone such as dimethicone or the more traditional gripe water can be helpful.

Pharmacists should remember the stress which is caused to mothers by a crying baby and endeavour to reassure mothers that crying is not always prompted by hunger pangs. The mother should also be advised to listen for unusual kinds of crying and reminded that crying babies can often be pacified by cuddling, speaking, and singing as well as by feeding.

10.2.5 Drinks between feeds

Boiled, cooled water (unsweetened) can be given or one of the ranges of baby drinks and fruit juices. Mothers should be encouraged to watch labels closely and to buy low-sugar varieties.

10.2.6 Weaning

Between the ages of four and six months, babies are generally ready to move on to solid foods in addition to their milk. Weaning should not take place before four months, because evidence from research suggests that early weaning may result in a greater likelihood of allergies. Some experts suggest that rice is a good first weaning food rather than wheat-based cereals and all weaning foods should be gluten-free.

10.2.7 Diarrhoea and vomiting

Rehydration therapy is now the only treatment recommended for diarrhoea and vomiting in infants and young children. The risks of dehydration mean that fluid and electrolyte intake are critical. Babies aged under one year who have vomiting and diarrhoea should always be referred to the GP, although rehydration therapy can be started. For children over one year, referral is advisable if the condition continues for longer than 24 hours or worsens in the meantime. Again, rehydration sachets should be given.

10.2.8 Responding to symptoms in babies

Pharmacists would be well advised to take great care in recommending medicines for young babies. Indeed, some would counsel no medicines should be advised at all during the first year of life. Bearing in mind the possible hazards of prescribing medicines for young babies (for example, rapid dehydration occurring in diarrhoea and infections, abdominal pain of unknown cause, changes in crying patterns, and so on), the possible complications and difficulty in establishing the cause of some symptoms means that great care should be exercised by pharmacists and their staff.

10.2.9 Vitamin supplements

The most recent government report on vitamin supplementation for infants recommended that all babies from the age of six months to two years who are not receiving breast or formula milk, and preferably up to five years old, should receive multi-vitamin supplements.

Mothers attending a baby clinic will be advised about vitamin supplementation. Vitamin drops can be bought at Well Baby clinics at reduced price. Mothers who visit the pharmacy can be asked whether vitamin drops are being given. If not, they can be obtained either from the baby clinic on prescription from the GP or purchased over the counter.

For older children, parents are often concerned at what they consider to be faddy eating habits and think that their children may be vitamin-deficient. Hence, they often ask pharmacists for suitable vitamin products. The pharmacist can encourage the keeping of a food diary to assess what is actually eaten by the child so that recommendations can be made about important foods to be added. The pharmacist can also enquire about the child's weight and general development to ascertain whether these are within normal limits. If the child is seriously underweight, they will need more than vitamins. Very often it is the case that parents are needlessly anxious about the tension which is associated with mealtimes by a child who refuses to eat particular foods. In addition, television and magazine advertising suggest that all children will benefit from vitamin supplementation.

In recent years this tendency has been exacerbated by the claimed benefit of vitamins in improving the IQ of children. On current evidence, routine vitamin supplementation for children cannot be recommended unless the food diary indicates that vitamin deficiency is likely. Further studies are currently being carried out to provide definitive data on vitamin and mineral supplementation and intelligence.

10.3 General dietary advice

The modified diet recommended by COMA and NACNE should not be followed in its entirety for young children. While there is much evidence that children receive far more saturated fat than is ideal, and this should be reduced, there is no recommendation that children should receive a large quantity of fibre. The danger is that, in their smaller gut, the increased fibre is likely to result in reduced appetite, with the possible consequence that they will not eat sufficient to prevent malnourishment. In addition, fibre can reduce the absorption of some vitamins. Most experts would agree that for children of twelve and under, a sensible approach would be to gradually reduce the calories obtained from fat between the ages of two and five. Fibre can gradually and slowly be increased from this age.

The best guide is weight and general fitness. Underweight children may have serious eating problems, but they may also have too much fibre in their diet, so that they become full too quickly and are not taking in sufficient calories. Overweight children should not be given sweet snacks between meals and their diet should be adjusted to include less sugar and fat.

10.4 Sugar and dental caries

Wherever possible in responding to symptoms for children, the pharmacist should recommend a sugar-free medicine; for most therapeutic uses, sugar-free formulations are now available. Many pharmacies stock and sell items of confectionery—for example barley sugar sticks and sweets—and such a policy is incompatible with prevention of dental caries and a health promotion image for the pharmacist.

From the weaning stage, parents should not add sugar and salt to food. If sweets are to be given to children, they are best eaten immediately after a meal, and the teeth brushed afterwards. Babies and children who wake during the night should be given water (boiled and cooled first, in the case of babies).

10.5 Head lice

Pharmacists are commonly asked to recommend prophylaxis and treatment for head lice. There is no such thing as effective prevention, and a better approach is to encourage regular examination of the child's hair. Indeed, it is thought that the use of insecticidal shampoos and lotions in an attempt to prevent infestation can enhance the resistance of lice, since they may be able to process small quantities of the insecticides. Accordingly, products should only be recommended when treatment is needed and, since most districts currently operate a rotational policy of carbaryl and malathion, the pharmacist should recommend the insecticide that is currently favoured.

While parents often prefer shampoo formulations, since these are more familiar, lotions (of carbaryl and malathion) provide a more effective treatment as the concentration of insecticide on the hair is much greater. In other words, since the lotion is left to dry on the hair, the insecticide is in contact with the hair and scalp for a longer period of time whereas, if a shampoo formulation is used, repeated treatments are needed at three-day intervals, and thus compliance may be low and might lead to reinfestation. One shampoo formulation containing a recently-introduced ingredient—phenothrin—is licensed for single-application use. Experts consider that two hours' treatment with a lotion is insufficient and advise that the lotion is left on overnight.

Both carbaryl and malathion are inactivated by heat, and parents should be advised that the hair should be left to dry naturally rather than subjected to a hair-dryer or dried close to a gas fire. Similarly, both insecticides are inactivated by chlorine in swimming pools and, if the child has been swimming before treatment, the hair should be thoroughly shampooed before the insecticide is applied.

Recently, new preparations containing pyrethroids have become available as a shampoo and a creme rinse. These insecticides are effective against both live lice and eggs and are not inactivated by heat or chlorine. Some districts have incorporated these new products into their rotation schedules and pharmacists can contact their District Pharmaceutical Officer to determine what their local policy is.

Since infestation spreads quickly through close contact, and symptoms do not become apparent until several hundred insect bites have been suffered, the current recommendation is that all family members are treated at the same time. Parents sometimes think that treatment failure has occurred because the empty egg shells, or nits, can still be seen in the hair as white, opalescent particles. These are firmly attached to the hair shaft and will not be removed simply by shampooing the hair. The use of a fine tooth-comb will facilitate removal of the nits; such a comb is more easily used on wet rather than dry hair.

Resistance to the two insecticides most commonly used is very rare, and treatment failure is more likely to be due to incorrect use of the product or to rapid reinfestation—back at school for example. Well-intentioned but misinformed letters from school headmasters advising the use of particular products can be countered by a telephone call from the pharmacist to explain the current thinking and policy.

The long association of head lice with poor hygiene is totally inaccurate. There is a major role for the pharmacist in reassuring anxious parents that head lice infestation is almost endemic amongst schoolchildren and that there is no stigma attached to the infection. Talks to local schoolchildren and staff can help to correct misapprehensions.

10.6 Threadworms

Like head lice, the subject of threadworm infestation is the cause of much anxiety and distress both to children and their parents. It has been estimated that, at any one time, between 20 and 30 per cent of schoolchildren aged under 10 years will be infected with thread-worms. The characteristic appearance of these worms has led to their name, and in fact the worms resemble small threads of white cotton which can readily be seen in the faeces or around the anus. The infection is transferred by eggs which are commonly found under the fingernails. They are swallowed after finger-sucking or nail-biting and then move into the gastrointestinal tract, finally hatching in the lower portion of the large bowel. At night, the female worms emerge to lay eggs on the perianal skin, and these eggs are secreted in a sticky, glue-like substance which is respons-ible for the symptom itch. The skin is scratched, more eggs are transferred under the fingernails, and the cycle begins all over again.

Treatment consists of anthelmintics such as mebendazole ('Ovex') or piperazine ('Pripsen'), both of which are available over the counter. Such treatment will not in itself prevent reinfestation, and practical advice should be offered aimed at breaking the cycle.

Advice on this subject should include keeping the fingernails short, the wearing of pyjamas in bed, having a warm bath after getting up in the morning (this helps to wash away the newly-laid eggs), and thorough cleaning of the nails using a nailbrush. Current thinking is that all family members should be treated at the same time, since symptoms may not manifest themselves for some time after the initial infestation takes place.

Threadworms are a common problem which will rarely need medical advice or treatment and can effectively be dealt with by the pharmacist.

10.7 Bedwetting

Parents sometimes ask pharmacists for advice and treatment for bedwetting (nocturnal enuresis). The pharmacist should be aware of the normal pattern and development of bladder control in children and of the reassuring statistics which can be offered to worried parents. One large study found that one in twenty children aged seven wet the bed at least once a week; by the age of ten, only one in forty children do so. Betwetting is commoner among boys than girls. Recent life changes such as starting school or being in hospital can induce enuresis in a child who has become dry. Pharmacists should be alert for symptoms of urinary tract infections which may sometimes precipitate a problem of bedwetting.

There is a variety of mechanical aids and alarms which are intended to awaken the child as soon as the first drops of urine are passed in order to prompt him to go to the toilet. In recent years these devices have become much more sophisticated and acceptable to parent and child. Child psychologists who have dealt with the problem of bedwetting are agreed that a system of small rewards is an effective means of encouraging 'dryness', whereas disapproval and punishments have the opposite to the desired effect.

A medical referral should be made, since further investigations and drug treatment may need to be initiated. Medical referral should also be advised if the pharmacist suspects that a urinary tract infection may be the cause of the problem. Some school nurses have bed alarms which can be loaned for a three-month trial period via the GP, who monitors progress. The pharmacist could investigate which, if any, of the local schools have this facility.

10.8 Childhood infections and antibiotics

Parents sometimes expect the GP to prescribe antibiotics for a child who has an upper respiratory tract or ear infection. They occasionally complain to the pharmacist that their child has not received the treatment he or she needs, and the pharmacist has an important role in explaining the difference between viral and bacterial infections in simple terms and in outlining those circumstances where antibiotic treatment is not warranted. Parental concern is often that their child is not getting the best treatment, and an explanation and reassurance from the pharmacist can be invaluable.

10.9 Case studies

'I've had a letter about his vaccinations—but they can be dangerous, can't they?'

A young mother who was a regular customer asked this question in response to the pharmacist's enquiry about the health of her recently-born baby. The baby is now three months old and should have had his first dose of diphtheria, pertussis, and polio vaccine last month. The pharmacist asked 'What makes you think that vaccinations are dangerous?' and the woman replied that she had heard about babies having brain damage afterwards. Giving the woman a copy of a leaflet about infant vaccinations, the pharmacist explained that there appeared to be a very small chance of brain damage from the whooping cough element of the vaccine. However, she went on, the modern vaccine is very highly purified and less likely to cause such problems. It was important to bear in mind, she said, that there is a far greater chance of brain damage as a result of whooping cough itself, especially in babies under six months old. She suggested that the woman should talk to her GP or health visitor before making a final decision.

'What's the best milk for babies?'

The customer who asked this question was a young woman, aged about 18. She was not a regular visitor to the pharmacy, and the pharmacist asked her about the baby. The child was hers and was now two weeks old. She had tried breast feeding but it 'didn't work', and in any case she didn't like it. The pharmacist asked if there had been any specific problem with breast-feeding and the young woman explained that the baby didn't take much milk and never seemed satisfied. She had bought some SMA Gold Cap last week and was giving the baby that, but wondered if it was the best milk. The pharmacist suggested that the milk was OK for a new baby and that the young woman might have a chat with the health visitor and perhaps have another try at breast-feeding. He explained that the health visitor would be able to help and give advice.

'I've read that vitamins make children more intelligent. Which ones do you think would be best? My children certainly need them!'

A customer with children aged six and eight had read in the daily paper that vitamins could make children cleverer. The pharmacist asked about their usual daily diet and the woman explained that she had been worried for months about their faddy eating. She said they rarely ate 'proper' meals but preferred crisps, biscuits, and fizzy pop. They refused point-blank to eat vegetables and only ate fruit very occasionally. The pharmacist explained that there was a lot of argument about vitamins and intelligence and that there was no agreement that the two were linked. However, if she was worried about the children's diet not giving enough vitamins, a daily multivitamin could help, he said. He wasn't promising any miracles as far as their intelligence was concerned but felt it could be helpful to supplement their vitamin intake.

'There's nits going around at the school. My children haven't got them but what have you got to make sure they don't?'

The pharmacist's heart sank on hearing this question—a common one. She explained that shampoos and lotions for treating head lice didn't work in preventing them. A better way, she said, was to comb the children's hair with a fine toothcomb. The hair could be examined too—paying particular attention to the nape of the neck, under the fringe, and behind the ears. If the children were infected, white empty eggshells (nits) would be seen on the hair, and tiny eggs closer to the scalp which take on the colour of the hair and were waiting to hatch out. Then a treatment would be needed. The woman was not convinced, because her mother always washed her hair with nit shampoo once a week and she never caught nits. The pharmacist explained again that the treatments were useless in preventing head lice and might not work so well if the child caught head lice later. She used a leaflet in the second explanation to emphasise the points she was making, and the customer finally accepted her explanation.

'My son's six and still wets the bed at night—have you got any medicine to stop it?'

The pharmacist asked whether the child had always wet the bed— the woman said no, from the age of about five he had been dry at night. The pharmacist then asked if anything had happened or if there had been any changes recently which might have been upsetting to the child. The woman explained that they had recently moved house and the boy had started at a new school.

The pharmacist explained that medicines were not used so often these days for bedwetting. It was quite a common problem, he said, especially if there had been a recent event like moving house. He advised the woman to take her son to the GP, just to get a check up. He said the GP might suggest a special alarm to be used at night and which had a very high success rate. The pharmacist gave the woman a leaflet published by the Enuresis Research and Information Centre (ERIC) and suggested she read it before taking the child to the GP so that she could find out a little more about the problem.

'My baby's got an awful cough and the doctor won't give her antibiotics—can you give her some?'

Firstly the pharmacist explained that, although antibiotics were very useful medicines, they didn't work in all infections. She asked if the doctor had seen and examined the child—he had. She then asked why the mother thought it was so important to have antibiotics. The woman explained that her previous doctor had always given them when any of the children had a cough. The pharmacist was conscious of the need not to impair the woman's confidence in either of the two prescribers. She briefly explained in simple terms about viruses and bacteria and that we now know that many infections are caused by viruses, where antibiotics don't work. She went on to say that, because the doctor had examined the child, he had made sure that antibiotics weren't needed. Finally she suggested some simple practical measures like using steam in the bedroom to humidify the air (by boiling a kettle for ten to fifteen minutes in there before the baby was put to bed) and suggested that a soothing mixture like 'Paediatric Simple Linctus' may also help.

11   Family planning and women's health

Traditionally, the pharmacy has always been a major outlet for the sale and supply of contraceptives. Given the problems of privacy in the pharmacy, the number of people who ask directly for advice about family planning is relatively small. However, the pharmacy is a good point from which to distribute information, in the form of leaflets, about contraceptive methods and about safer sex in relation to AIDS. The availability of such leaflets, together with the generally reduced extent to which Family Planning Clinics operate in some areas because of financial cuts within the NHS, mean that the community pharmacist may well be asked for advice on a greater number of occasions in the future. It is, therefore, vitally important that the pharmacist is well informed about contraceptive methods and about pregnancy and ovulation testing. Women often consult their pharmacist and ask for advice and treatment for conditions such as vaginal thrush and cystitis. In addition to over-the-counter treatment, where appropriate, the pharmacist is in a good position to offer practical self-help advice to prevent future occurrences of these conditions.

In this chapter we will consider the main methods of contraception and the types of questions which pharmacy clients may ask about them. We will then go on to look at aspects of women's health which may generate questions in the pharmacy.

11.1 Contraceptive methods

Essentially, there are six main forms of contraception.

- Oral contraceptive pills
- Barrier methods
- Intra-uterine devices (previously known as 'the coil')

- Injectables
- 'Natural' birth-control
- Female sterilization and vasectomy

11.1.1 Oral contraceptives

Oral contraceptives are of two main types: the combined oral contraceptive and the progestogen-only pill.

The combined oral contraceptive

The combined oral contraceptive is highly effective against pregnancy and works mainly by suppressing ovulation. Failure rates vary between less than 1 pregnancy per 100 woman years (0.1 to 7 per cent) depending on how well it is taken. Over the years, the relative doses of oestrogen and progestogen in the combined pill have been reduced. Most products require the pill to be taken for three weeks, with a one week break in which a withdrawal bleed occurs. There has been a great deal of publicity about adverse effects from the pill, and in particular there has been concern about the dose of oestrogen contained in it. A pill with the lowest possible effective dose of oestrogen is now prescribed. Taking the combined oral contraceptive pill gives a protective effect against ovarian cancer and endometrial cancer and fibroids. Use of the combined pill has, however, been linked to an increased risk of developing heart disease and a possible increased risk of breast cancer and cervical cancer. Additionally, and in very rare cases, combined pill use has been linked to cancer of the liver. The risk/benefit ratio of taking the combined pill must be carefully considered by the woman and her prescriber. The risks of circulatory problems and, in particular, cerebrovascular events are greatly increased in women of all ages who smoke and those in older age groups. For women who are aged 35 or over and are smokers the combined pill should be discontinued. In non-smokers, the combined pill can be continued until at least the age of 45. Pharmacists should be aware that migraine-type headaches in women taking the combined pill can sometimes be a warning of adverse cerebrovascular changes. Such women should be referred to their doctor.

Drugs such as rifampicin and phenytoin, which induce liver

enzymes, may speed up metabolism of oestrogen and progestogen and make the pill ineffective. More controversial is the interaction between the pill and antibiotics. Here broad spectrum antibiotics disturb the bacterial flora of the gut and prevent the reabsorption of oestrogen. The effect is on oestrogen not progestogen, and ampicillin and tetracyclines are the drugs most commonly cited. Additional contraceptive precautions would be wise. Low-dose tetracyclines in acne are reported not to cause problems. Prolonged or severe diarrhoea and vomiting may render the combined pill less effective; diarrhoea may occur as an adverse effect from a broad-spectrum antibiotic. If the woman has diarrhoea and vomiting, either in association with an antibiotic or independently, additional precautions should be taken for as long as the diarrhoea lasts and for seven days afterwards.

The progestogen-only pill

The progestogen-only pill (mini-pill) must be taken regularly and at the same time each day and requires a high degree of patient motivation. This pill is taken every day without a break and each pill gives 27 hours' protection. This method of contraception works mainly by altering the production of cervical mucus, which in turn makes it difficult for sperm to reach the egg and enable fertilization, and also by stopping ovulation in some 40 per cent of cycles. The effect of the mini-pill on the penetrability of cervical mucus is at its minimum each time a dose is taken. Many women who take the progestogen-only pill experience irregular periods and break-through bleeding, although their cycle often becomes more regular with longer-term use. Some women find that their periods become lighter and others have no periods at all.

The progestogen-only pill has a relatively higher failure rate than does the combined pill (1–4 per cent). As we have said, the pill should be taken at the same time each day. If it is delayed by longer than three hours, contraceptive protection may be lost. Broad spectrum antibiotics do not interact with the progestogen-only pill but enzyme inducers do.

'Missed' pills

Women sometimes consult the pharmacist, explaining that they have 'missed' a pill and asking if they might be pregnant or whether they should use additional contraceptive methods. The advice recommended by the Family Planning Association is as follows.

For combined pills:

If you forget a pill, take it as soon as you remember, and the next one at your normal time. If you are 12 or more hours late with any pill (especially the first or last in the packet), the pill may not work. As soon as you remember, continue normal pill-taking. However, you will not be protected for the next 7 days and must either not have sex or use another method, such as the condom. If these 7 days run beyond the end of your packet, start the next packet at once, when you have finished the present one, i.e., do not have a time interval between packets. This will mean you may not have a period until the end of 2 packets but this does you no harm. Nor does it matter if you see some bleeding on pill-taking days. If you are using every day (ED) pills, miss out the 7 inactive pills. If you are not sure which these are, ask your doctor.

For the progestogen-only pill:

If you forget a pill, take it as soon as you remember, and carry on with the next pill at the right time. If the pill is more than three hours overdue, you are not protected. Continue normal pill-taking but you must also use another method, such as the condom, for the next 48 hours. If you have vomiting, or very severe diarrhoea, the pill may not work. Continue to take it, but you may not be protected from the first day of vomiting or diarrhoea. Use another method, such as the condom, for any intercourse during the stomach upset and for the next 48 hours.

Emergency contraception

It should be noted that there is a third use for the pill, namely emergency contraception (post-coital contraception; formerly known as the 'morning-after pill'). The emergency hormonal method is a special dose of combined pill used after unprotected sex or if a method has not worked—for example, a burst condom. Usually, a combined oestrogen/progestogen preparation is used (250 mcg levonorgestrel, 50 mcg ethinyloestradiol). Two tablets are taken immediately, two tablets after twelve hours. The treatment must be initiated within three days of having unprotected sex, but the earlier the better. The method is effective but the high dose of oestrogen which is consumed may cause nausea and even vomiting. Following post-coital contraception, the woman's period may begin on time or a little earlier or later than anticipated. The efficacy of this method is 96–99 per cent.

Pharmacists have occasionally been asked to supply post-coital contraception as an 'emergency supply'. While such a supply may be made under the provisions of the Medicines Act, it is a matter of the pharmacist's own professional judgment as to whether this course of action should be taken. The Royal Pharmaceutical Society's Law Department reminds pharmacists of the requirements for such a supply: they are that the pharmacist must establish that the patient has been prescribed the treatment on a previous occasion. The pharmacist should also attempt to contact the prescriber in order to confirm the supply. If this is not possible, the pharmacist should strongly advise the patient to inform the prescriber of the supply. With the patient's agreement, the pharmacist may later inform the prescriber that the emergency supply was made. Such a request for a supply of emergency hormonal contraception places the pharmacist in a difficult professional situation, since the treatment will only be effective if given within 72 hours of unprotected intercourse.

If, as has actually happened in practice, the supply was requested on a Saturday morning following unprotected intercourse the previous evening, when the local surgery was not due to open for appointments again until Monday, the 72-hour period might theoretically elapse before treatment could be obtained. Family Planning Clinic doctors also prescribe emergency hormonal contraception and a woman may attend any such clinic which is open.

In an alternative form of post-coital birth control, an intrauterine device (IUD) is fitted. The device should be fitted as soon as possible after unprotected intercourse, and within five days of the calculated date of ovulation. However, IUDs are not suitable for all women, and thus this method of emergency contraception is used relatively rarely.

11.1.2 Barrier methods

Condoms (Sheath)

The increasing incidence of AIDS and other sexually-transmitted diseases has meant that, in recent years, the use of condoms has seen a revival in popularity. Estimates suggest that sales of condoms have been increasing at the rate of 20 per cent per year since 1983 among the homosexual as well as the heterosexual community. The use of condoms is a central feature of advice on safer sex. Only those condoms which have BSI (British Standards Institute) 'Kite-mark' approval should be stocked, since these will have been tested to meet a particular standard. People who buy condoms will some-times also wish to purchase a spermicidal gel or lubricant, and all the spermicides currently on the market are compatible with condoms. The pharmacist should advise that, whilst water-based lubricants can be used, oil-based products are incompatible, so that petroleum jelly and baby or other oils should not be used with condoms. Present figures for the contraceptive-effectiveness of condoms show 85–98 per cent reliability. It is important to dispel the myth that condoms are not effective; condoms can only be as good as their user.

Caps and diaphragms

These prevent the passage of sperm into the womb. The cervical cap is held in place by suction and comes in three shapes and in a variety of sizes. Prescribing of these is best done at a Family Planning Clinic, as is also the case with diaphragms. The diaphragm is also made of rubber but is kept in place by a pliable metal rim which is covered in rubber. If a woman complains of discomfort from a cap or diaphragm, refitting may be needed. Caps and diaphragms also provide some protection against sexually-transmitted diseases and appear to protect women from cancer of the cervix.

A spermicide must be used with cap and diaphragm alike and the device should be left in place for a least six hours after intercourse but removed within 24 hours. Contrary to popular opinion, the diaphragm can be inserted any time before intercourse. If, however, intercourse occurs more than three hours after inserting the diaphragm then a further application of spermicide should be used.

The Family Planning Clinic will give advice about cleaning caps. General rules to be followed are that unscented soap should be used in order to prevent irritant reactions and that the device should be left to dry. Caps and diaphragms should not be boiled, nor should they be cleaned with disinfectant, bleach, detergent, or any other chemical. Family planning advisors suggest that cap users should visit their Family Planning Clinic at six-monthly intervals (or sooner if the woman is experiencing any problems) to check that the size is still correct. The reason for this is that, if the body weight changes by more than 3 kg (7 lbs), a different size of cap may be needed. A woman who has recently had a baby, miscarriage, or abortion will also probably require a different size.

Used carefully, caps and diaphragms can provide a high rate of contraceptive effectiveness (85–98 per cent) and—as indicated earlier—good advice is that a spermicide should also be used. Since these devices are made of rubber, the same principles apply in the use of spermicides, which should always be water-based.

The contraceptive vaginal sponge

This is made from polyurethane foam and contains a spermicide. As a method of contraception, it is less reliable than other barrier methods and much less effective than the oral contraceptive pill. In an average year, for every 100 women using the sponge carefully and consistently, 9 become pregnant: with less careful use, the figure can rise to between 9 and 25. Family planning experts suggest that this method should not be used by itself if avoiding pregnancy is absolutely essential. It may be more suitable for women whose fertility is reduced—for example those aged over 45. The sponge should be moistened with water before insertion and will then remain effective for 24 hours. As with the cap or diaphragm, the sponge must be left in place for at least six hours after intercourse, so it may be kept in the vagina for up to 30 hours.

11.1.3 Intra-uterine devices (IUDs)

IUDs are fitted into the uterus and usually consist of a plastic moulding which is coated with thin copper wire. Advantages of the method are that it is effective immediately after insertion and provides long-term protection. The Family Planning Association's current policy is that intra-uterine contraceptive devices need not generally be changed more often than every five years and the contraceptive efficacy of some devices has been shown to be far longer than five years.

However, IUDs are not suitable for all women. Sometimes the

IUD is expelled soon after insertion. The main problem with the device, however, is that it may tend to cause heavier, longer, and more painful periods in some women. Women who use the IUD as their method of contraception can be more prone to infections in the uterus and fallopian tubes—pelvic inflammatory disease ('PID')—particularly if they or their partner are not sexually faithful to each other.

The IUD is not usually recommended as a method of contraception for young women who have not had children. Generally, the IUD will need to be replaced about every five years. It is recommended that, about six weeks after insertion, an examination should be made to ensure that the IUD is sited correctly and there are no problems.

While women with an IUD fitted will sometimes experience painful periods, symptoms which suggest infection or pelvic inflammatory disease—severe pain at times other than menstruation, or signs of systemic infection such as feverishness, or vaginal discharge—would indicate immediate referral to the doctor.

11.1.4 Injectables

Injectable contraceptives contain progestogens and are usually given as 'depot' formulations which will have a long-term action. Of the two products which are currently used in the UK, injections are needed at 8-weekly ('Noristerat') or 12-weekly ('Depo-Provera') intervals. Advantages of this form of contraception are its effectiveness, which is at an extremely high rate (less than 1 per cent failure), and that the method does not rely on memory, unlike pill-taking. However, side-effects are common. Some women find they have fewer periods and some become amenorrhoeic and have no periods at all. Others find their periods become heavier, at least initially. Weight-gain and depression have been reported as side-effects of this method of contraception. Injectable contraceptives are less effective in obese women than in women of normal weight.

Injectable methods are generally not recommended for women who wish to start a family in the near future, since their effect is cumulative and, even after stopping the injections, it may be a minimum of 9–10 months or longer before pregnancy is achieved.

11.1.5 Natural methods

Natural methods of contraception (formerly known as the 'rhythm' method) are based on the signs and symptoms in the body which indicate ovulation and therefore the fertile time. Becoming familiar with how natural family planning works allows a couple to either plan a pregnancy or avoid conception. The methods therefore involve careful recording of the signs and the keeping of records. The fertile period lasts for some seven days—five days before ovulation and at least two days afterwards—since sperm are viable for up to five days in the vagina. There are a number of different natural family planning methods which will allow a woman to observe the naturally-occurring signs and symptoms of the fertile and infertile phases of the menstrual cycle.

If natural family planning is practised by a highly-motivated couple who are well taught and committed to the method and will practise it carefully and conscientiously, then it is effective. Under such circumstances, of 100 women using the method for a year, only 2 will become pregnant (symptothermal method). Should the method not be carefully followed, the effectiveness is drastically reduced and 20 pregnancies are likely to result per 100 women per year.

Many pharmacies stock fertility thermometers and temperature recording charts, together with their instructions. If the woman has not received explanation of how to use the natural method of contraception, then the details need to be carefully outlined by the pharmacist and referral to a recognized centre teaching natural family planning is essential. A private area in the pharmacy is obviously desirable for such a consultation to take place.

11.1.6 Female sterilization and male vasectomy

Where a couple have completed their family or are sure that they do not want to have children, female sterilization or vasectomy for the male may be requested. For all practical purposes, these procedures should be regarded as irreversible. Occasionally, reversal operations are carried out but there are difficulties involved and the procedure may not be a success.

A vasectomy is carried out as a minor operation usually under local anaesthetic. After making small cuts in the scrotum, the vas deferens are cut and sealed. While sex can be resumed as soon as the discomfort has ceased, it is important that other methods of contraception are used initially. There may still be active sperm present, and semen tests are normally carried out to check for their presence. Two clear semen tests must be produced before the vasectomy becomes a totally effective method of contraception.

Female sterilization is a more invasive and larger operation than is a vasectomy and may involve a light general anaesthetic or a local anaesthetic. The fallopian tubes are either cut or blocked in order to prevent eggs travelling from the ovaries to the uterus. Following a female sterilization, additional contraceptive measures are usually advised until the next menstrual period.

11.2 Pregnancy and ovulation testing

For many years, pharmacies have provided a pregnancy testing service which has been widely used because of its accessibility and convenience. Additionally, home pregnancy testing kits are sold from pharmacies. With the increasing development of technology, the accuracy of pregnancy tests is now extremely high, and the tests provide clearer results. In offering a pregnancy testing service, the pharmacist must comply with the Royal Pharmaceutical Society's guidelines (see Chapter 5, p. 92). As with any other diagnostic or screening test, the product and method used must be of a high level of accuracy, and the pharmacist or member of staff who carries out the test must be trained in its use and interpretation of the results. The communication of the results of the test to the client must be done in an atmosphere of privacy and using great tact. Often the pharmacist has no way of knowing whether the woman might be desperate to have a child or whether becoming pregnant might be regarded as a disaster. Research in pharmacies shows that around two-thirds of women who buy a home pregnancy testing kit want the result to be positive and that the commonest age group of women buying such kits is between 25 and 34 years, these accounting for almost two-thirds of all pregnancy kits purchased.

11.2.1 Test accuracy

The development of monoclonal pregnancy tests has greatly increased the sensitivity of such tests. Essentially, the test detects the presence of human chorionic gonadotrophin (HCG). Such tiny amounts can now be detected that some pregnancy tests claim that a result can be obtained even before the first missed period. However, the pharmacist must remember that almost two-thirds of early pregnancies spontaneously miscarry within the first 20 days after implantation. In fact, what a woman might previously have thought to be a late period could indeed be an early pregnancy which has miscarried. For a woman who wanted to become pregnant, such a test result could only be distressing. For over-the-counter sale, a kit containing two tests will allow the woman to check her first result some time later or, alternatively, allows a second test to be carried out if a mistake has been made with the procedure in the first test.

11.2.2 Positive test results

For any pregnancy test which is performed in the pharmacy, if a positive result is obtained then the woman must be strongly advised to make an appointment to see her doctor. This will ensure that appointments are made at ante-natal clinics and that the woman is properly cared for during her pregnancy and also that she can be encouraged to make use of the health facilities available. Some women will not wish to continue their pregnancy and, again, medical help must be sought. If the woman was reluctant to consult her family doctor, she could be referred to one of the pregnancy charities such as the British Pregnancy Advisory Service for medical advice.

11.2.3 Negative test results

If a woman's period is more than five days late but the pregnancy test produces a negative result, the advice to be given should be to see her GP. The reason for this is that there may be a serious reason for the negative test result, such as an ectopic pregnancy, which may sometimes cause a false negative result. Ectopic pregnancies are more common in women who use the IUD as a form of contraception than in those who use other methods.

11.2.4 Ovulation prediction kits

Several brands of ovulation prediction kit are now available through pharmacies and these work by detecting a surge of luteinizing hormone (LH) which normally happens about 30 hours before the egg is released. The amount of time which elapses between the LH surge and ovulation may vary between 24 and 36 hours. By having intercourse during this time, the couple will know that they are maximizing their chances of conception.

The products involve a daily test around the time when ovulation is expected. This would usually be 14 days before the expected date of the next period, but even in women with regular cycles there may be a variation of 1 or 2 days either side of the expected time. For women who have irregular menstrual cycles, missing the LH surge can be a real problem. The self-test ovulation kits may also fail to be effective if the LH surge is very brief and falls between the once-daily tests or if the level of LH is very low. Where the LH surge is thought to be brief, twice-daily testing will increase the chances of detection, but this is, naturally, a more expensive procedure. Manufacturers of ovulation test kits recommend that any woman who does not conceive, or who fails to detect a surge of LH, after three menstrual cycles should go and see her GP for further discussions and investigations.

For the future, it may be that pharmacies will choose to offer an ovulation prediction test service, where urine samples will be brought in by the client for in-pharmacy testing on a daily basis. While this development appears not to have occurred to date, it is an alternative to self-testing kits and may be suitable for some women who do not feel confident about using such a kit.

11.3 Women's health

Women form the majority of customers in community pharmacies. Hence, it is important for the pharmacist to have an awareness of common conditions about which women may seek advice and treatment. In this section we will consider some of the commonest conditions which women are known to ask about in pharmacies and the practical advice which can be offered.

11.3.1 Cystitis

This is a common condition in which passing urine produces a painful burning sensation and where the urge to pass urine occurs very frequently when, in fact, there is little to be voided. Although some cases of cystitis are due to bacterial infection, a significant proportion have no apparent cause. Some women suffer from recurrent bouts which may be induced by irritants such as perfumed bubble baths and talcum powders, the rubber from which condoms are made, or other contraceptive products such as spermicides, caps, or diaphragms. Intercourse itself can induce the symptoms of cystitis if damage to the urethra occurs, and 'honeymoon cystitis' is quite common in young women.

In general, self-help measures for cystitis can be useful. Over-the-counter treatments are based on potassium or sodium citrate which makes the urine more alkaline. In cystitis the urine is acidic and this is part of the reason why its passage is painful. Thus, to alkalinize the urine reduces discomfort. Bacteria are less able to live in an alkaline medium, so this effect, too, can be helpful. Pregnant women with the symptoms of cystitis should never be advised to try self-treatment, since untreated urinary tract infections in pregnancy may lead to serious kidney problems. Signs of infection—such as fever, loin pain, and cloudy or smelly urine—would be indications for immediate referral rather than self-treatment. For women in whom cystitis is a recurrent problem, self-help books such as Angela Kilmartin's *Understanding cystitis* can be extremely valuable.

11.3.2 Vaginal thrush

Some women are prone to recurrent attacks of this infection, which often produces intense vaginal itching and a creamy white discharge. Predisposing factors include the use of wide spectrum oral antibiotics which alter the balance of the normal bacterial flora and make conditions easier for the yeast (*Candida*) to grow. Pregnant women are more prone to vaginal thrush because of hormonal changes. And diabetics—either undiagnosed or those in whom diabetes is not controlled—are prone because sugar in the urine provides nutrients on which the yeast can feed. Unexplained recurrent attacks of thrush may be an early sign of diabetes: if the condition is combined with other symptoms such as weight loss, increasing thirst, and increasing passage of urine, the woman should immediately be referred to her doctor. Self-treatment of vaginal thrush is currently difficult, since the most effective treatments— that is to say, vaginal pessaries—are not available over the counter but must be obtained on prescription. Anti-fungal creams can be purchased over the counter and may be a useful self-treatment until an appointment with the doctor can be made.

Self-help measures for thrush include the wearing of cotton (rather than nylon) underwear to allow the evaporation of perspiration, and taking care to wipe from front to back after defecation to prevent transmission of the yeast from the bowel to the vagina. Self-treatment with live yoghurt has been recommended, since the lactic acid produced by the lactobacillus will help to acidify the vaginal environment and make it more difficult for the yeast to grow. Women who want to try this treatment may insert a small amount of yoghurt using a tampon.

11.3.3 Menstrual problems

It is estimated that one in two menstruating women suffer from dysmenorrhoea (period pains) and an even higher proportion from the premenstrual syndrome ('PMS') in a mild to severe form. Dysmenorrhoea can be beneficially treated with over-the-counter analgesics of which ibuprofen is the most effective, providing there are no contra-indications to its use. Pain at times of the cycle other than menstruation should be regarded with suspicion and will require referral. PMS occurs when cyclical symptoms are experienced after ovulation in that part of the menstrual cycle which precedes the actual period. Such symptoms can be both physical (of which the commonest is breast tenderness) and emotional (including irritability and tiredness). Some studies have shown evening primrose oil to be effective in breast tenderness, while vitamin B6 (pyridoxine) at a dose of 50 mg per day has been shown to mitigate irritability, depression and fatigue in PMS in some women.

11.3.4 Menopausal problems

A common problem for menopausal and post-menopausal women is vaginal dryness, which can make sexual intercourse uncomfortable and even painful. This is due to hormonal changes which result in natural vaginal lubrication becoming reduced. Over-the-counter products can be purchased in the form of simple lubricants such as 'KY Jelly' and the long-acting 'Replens'. If such treatment is not successful, the woman should be referred to her doctor, who may prescribe an oestrogen vaginal cream which will correct the symptoms.

Pharmacists are sometimes asked by women about the effectiveness and safety of hormone replacement therapy (HRT) following the menopause. Research shows that the majority of women are aware of HRT, most of them through the media. Many are also aware of the much-publicized, potentially increased risk of breast cancer from HRT. Current thinking is that the benefits of hormone replacement therapy include a protective effect against the development of osteoporosis and heart disease, while the risks include a slight increase in the incidence of breast cancer after long-term use. On a statistical basis, the woman is far more likely to suffer from osteoporosis or heart disease than from breast cancer. However, the pharmacist can offer this information and enable an informed choice to be made.

Osteoporosis is a condition which is common in elderly women and results from the loss of bone mass. Supplementing dietary calcium is of little value and, following the menopause, hormonal therapy is needed to maintain bone density. Exercise can also maintain bone density but must be started at an early age—that is, before the age of 30 years—for maximum benefit and carried out on a regular basis. Regular exercise also has beneficial protective effects on the heart and can be recommended for women of all ages. Swimming and walking are both excellent forms of exercise for the pharmacist to advise.

11.4 Case studies

An anxious-looking young woman aged around twenty-five asks to speak to the pharmacist. She says that she forgot to take her pill yesterday—could she become pregnant?

The pharmacist invited the woman to a quiet part of the shop where their conversation could be held in some privacy. After asking which pill the woman took and determining that a combined oral contraceptive was involved and that the woman was halfway through the pack, the pharmacist asked exactly what had happened. The woman explained that she normally took her pill first thing each morning. Yesterday, though, she forgot and did not realize until this morning. She took both pills together and hoped that would be OK. The pharmacist explained that missing pills at the beginning or near the end of the pack are the most crucial. It was unlikely that the woman would become pregnant. He advised the woman to use additional contraceptive measures for seven days and suggested using the condom together with a spermicide.

A young woman was looking at the display of contraceptives on the medicines counter and picked up a pack of vaginal sponges. After waiting until the shop was empty she asked the counter assistant if the sponges worked. The counter assistant asked the pharmacist to deal with the query.

The pharmacist asked if any other method of contraception was being used. The woman explained that she had been taking the pill until quite recently but that her doctor suggested she come off it because she was a heavy smoker—he had prescribed the progestogen-only pill instead. She is due to start taking the progestogen-only pill next week and her doctor has advised that she use an additional method of contraception for the first 48 hours. The pharmacist advises that the condom plus spermicide is a more reliable contraceptive method than is the sponge and, after asking whether the woman needs any further information about the progestogen-only pill, finds she is unsure about how to take it. The pharmacist shows the woman a leaflet about this method of contraception and explains that the new pill is to be taken at the same time each day, and should be taken every day without a break. He suggests that the woman takes the leaflet away and reads it and comes back to see him if she has any other queries.

12 Drug misuse

In their everyday practice, pharmacists come across drug misuse in many forms, ranging from the use of prescription drugs for inappropriate lengths of time or at inappropriate dosages (for example, benzodiazepines) to the misuse of products which are available over-the-counter (such as codeine linctus) and the use of controlled drugs illegally—for example, via forged prescriptions. The knowledge base and interpersonal skills of the pharmacist are particularly crucial in dealing with drug misusers. A non-judgemental and professional approach is essential. Involvement with, and an awareness of, the requirements of problem drug users, including registered drug addicts, is also of importance. The pharmacist should liaise with local agencies dealing with drug misusers and work closely with them.

12.1 What is drug misuse?

The World Health Organization defines drug dependency in this way: 'A person is dependent on a drug or alcohol when it becomes very difficult or even impossible for him/her to stop taking the drug or alcohol without help, after having taken it regularly for some time. Dependence may be physical or psychological, or both'.

The perception of many people of a drug abuser or misuser is the antisocial and archetypal injecting heroin addict who leads a criminal lifestyle to support his habit. As pharmacists, we should disabuse ourselves of this image and be aware that the potential for drug misuse is far wider than this. There are three main categories:

1. illicit drug use;

2. misuse of prescription-only medicines;

3. misuse of over-the-counter medicines and other substances which may be legally purchased.

12.1.1 Illicit drug use

During this century, the control of drugs which are liable to misuse has become ever tighter in response to wider use in the community. In the nineteenth century the use of laudanum and other opiates began in the higher social classes and amongst the artistic community—for example, Coleridge, and de Quincey in *Confessions of an English opium eater*—and subsequently became widespread. Other famous 'users' were some of the English Pre-Raphaelites—for example, the poet and painter Dante Gabriel Rossetti. Concern at the effects of the extensive use of laudanum in society, and particularly at this being given to babies and small children, led to controls over distribution and sales.

The 1920s were years of experimentation with drugs such as hallucinogenic substances and cocaine among the intelligentsia. Perhaps the best known example is Aldous Huxley. In *Brave new world* he describes the heady brew called the 'soma', with its potential for political control over the masses. Huxley continued to experiment with drugs into at least the late 1940s and early 1950s with hallucinogens such as mescalin.

Drug misuse was reduced during the years of the Second World War but in the post-war era it increased, particularly in the 1960s—another time of experimentation. Some of the reasons for this increase were cheap supplies of drugs such as LSD, cross-cultural factors such as the 'Hippie Trail to India', the changing social climate, and a small but significant number of prescribers who were prepared to prescribe large quantities of drugs of misuse, especially amphetamine injections.

In response to this misuse of groups of medicines other than opiates, Parliament attempted to control the situation. It is interesting for young pharmacists to note that, 20 years ago, barbiturates were commonly prescribed as hypnotics and were not subject to any restrictions. Amphetamines were widely available for slimming purposes and benzedrine inhalers could be sold over-the-counter. It was only with the introduction and implementation of the 1968 Medicines Act that manufacturers of some over-the-counter products were required to review their formulations. Some of these contained relatively high doses of morphine, often in the form of 'chlorodyne' or tincture of chloroform and morphine.

Notification of drug misusers

A particular feature of legislation in the UK is the facility for drug addicts to be notified to the Home Office and to receive regular supplies of drugs on NHS prescription. An index of addicts was established to provide statistical information on narcotics abuse. The Misuse of Drugs (Notification of and Supply to Addicts) Regulations 1973 require doctors to notify addicts to the Home Office. Drugs for which such notification is required are shown in Table 12.1.

Prescribing of heroin, cocaine, and dipipanone to addicts for the treatment of addiction is limited to those doctors licensed by the Home Office to do so.

The scale of the problem

There were 14 785 notified drug addicts in the UK in 1989, and it is estimated that around one-quarter of community pharmacies are involved in dispensing for such patients. The number of *notified* drug misusers does not, of course, register the *true* number of people who misuse notifiable drugs, which was estimated at between 75 000 and 150 000 for 1986. These figures relate only to *notifiable* drugs, and therefore exclude other drugs such as cannabis and amphetamines. The 1986 estimates were that a further 75 000–150 000 people were misusers of non-notifiable drugs.

Legal classification of drugs of misuse

It has been argued that the results of the legislative process has been to move sections of society from legal to illegal drug use where use

Table 12.1   Notifiable drugs—Misuse of Drugs Regulations 1973

Cocaine	Methadone
Dextromoramide	Morphine
Diamorphine	Opium
Dipipanone†	Oxycodone
Hydrocodone	Pethidine
Hydromorphone	Phenazocine
Levorphanol	

† Added to the list in 1985

of a particular drug (for example, cannabis) is part of their cultural background. In the UK, controlled drugs are categorized into Classes A–C (on which penalties are based and Class A drugs dealt with most severely) and Schedules 1–5, which define the legal requirements for prescribing and supply.

Cannabis is subject to stringent restrictions in law and is the only illicit drug where there has been significant public support for its use to be legalized. In some countries—for example, Holland—cannabis use has effectively been decriminalized in an attempt to separate 'hard' and 'soft' drug use. Through the Dutch system cannabis is sold in coffee houses, which must be registered for that purpose, and who pay tax on sales. Should such outlets be found to also sell 'hard' drugs, their licence is revoked. Thus, possession of cannabis for the individual's own use is not a criminal offence in Holland, but penalties remain for those who sell from other than registered outlets. The Dutch programme's philosophy is to reduce demand and there has been a reduction in cannabis use since its introduction. In 17- and 18-year-olds usage fell from 10 per cent in 1976 to 6 per cent in 1986. The Dutch experience also appears to show that, by separating the supply of 'soft' and 'hard' drugs, the move from the former to the latter is less likely to occur.

Whilst it is relatively easy to place misused medicines under a tight regime of control, there is little political will to control other substances such as alcohol. In addition, there are grave practical difficulties in controlling widely-available materials such as solvents and aerosols, although the Intoxication Substances Supply Act 1985 protects the under-16s to some extent in this area. In the current situation, where the risk of catching HIV and developing AIDS from sharing injecting equipment and using dirty needles is large, pharmacists are increasingly being encouraged to sell or supply needles and syringes. It is acknowledged that the risk to the public from the spread of HIV overrides that presented by a possible proliferation of intravenous abusers. The issue of community pharmacists' involvement in reducing the spread of HIV by supplying needles and syringes, and by participating in needle exchange schemes, will be discussed later in the chapter.

12.1.2 Misuse of prescribed medicines

This group of drugs comprises those which are prescription-only medicines and which have a common medicinal use (in contrast to some of those described in the previous section—for example cocaine, which is rarely used for medicinal purposes, other than in eye and nasal drops).

Misuse of prescribed drugs can take several forms. Controlled drugs such as morphine may be sought by drug addicts. Whilst doctors, including GPs, are not allowed to prescribe for addiction unless they have a special licence, issued by the Home Office, they are still allowed to prescribe controlled drugs for their therapeutic uses, and drug misusers may persuade them of an urgent need—for example acute pain—or may simply pressurize the doctor to prescribe supplies. Pharmacists should be aware of the possibility of drug misuse by other health care personnel and should be alert, for example, to prescribers ordering large quantities of controlled drugs on signed orders, presenting signed orders for such drugs regularly, or regularly collecting supplies of prescribed controlled drugs on behalf of different patients. While such incidents are not common, the pharmacist should recognize that they have happened from time to time.

Other prescribed drugs which have the potential for dependence include benzodiazepines, to which 15–44 per cent of long-term patients become addicted. Concern over the effects of such long-term use of these drugs led to the issuing of a statement by the Committee of Safety of Medicines which recommends that they should not be prescribed for other than short-term use—normally a maximum period of four weeks. The Royal Pharmaceutical Society Council issued a statement to pharmacists on benzodiazepines in 1989, encouraging pharmacists to become more involved in counselling patients taking benzodiazepines and in discussions with the prescriber.

The legal implications of long-term prescribing of benzodiazepines are yet to be decided but hundreds of patients are currently involved in legal actions against prescribers. While pharmacists have not yet been involved in such litigation, the suggestion has been made that, by continuing to dispense benzodiazepine prescriptions without question, the pharmacist might be liable. Thus, benzodiazepines set a precedent for the future. The pharmacist can reiterate the doctor's advice that these drugs are valuable for short-term use. However, the pharmacist has a professional duty of care, and where there are known or anticipated side-effects from medium- to long-term use these should be acted upon.

Barbiturates are still misused, although their therapeutic use has fallen considerably during the last decade.

Forged prescriptions

Medicines and ethics—a guide for pharmacists contains guidance on detecting forged prescriptions. Confirming the prescriber's intentions is imperative where there is any suspicion on the pharmacist's part of a possible forgery. Telephone calls to prescribers should be made using a number obtained from the telephone directory or from Directory Inquiries and not from headed paper, as false letter-headings may be used. Occasionally, convincing forgeries of prescribers' details and telephone numbers have been made on FP10 prescriptions and the telephone number of the prescriber should therefore be checked.

Experience has shown that some factors have been associated with forged prescriptions and the pharmacist should be wary of prescriptions for drugs with potential for misuse:

- from unknown prescribers;

- from new patients;

- containing excessive quantities;

- where uncharacteristic prescribing or method of prescription-writing occurs from a known prescriber;

- where a letter-heading is compiled using 'Letraset' or similar methods;

- where the prescription states 'Dr' before or after the prescriber's signature.

The Royal Pharmaceutical Society's Law Department advises that pharmacists should apply these precautions to all prescriptions for drugs liable to misuse, and not simply to those for controlled drugs.

12.1.3 Over-the-counter products

All community pharmacists have been confronted with customers who wish to buy products which are known to be liable to misuse. The classic example is that of codeine linctus, but several other over-the-counter medicine ingredients are subject to misuse. There are both legal and ethical points concerned with the sale of such products. The pharmacist is under no legal obligation to sell any medicine to a customer and is entitled to refuse the sale of any medicine where possible misuse is suspected or known. While there is no legal requirement for pharmacists to keep records of such sales, the pharmacist is, however, required to keep invoices for those pharmacy medicines which fall under the CD Invoice category for at least two years. The Royal Pharmaceutical Society's' Code of Ethics, in its guidance notes, recommends that those over-the-counter medicines which are liable to abuse should be sold personally by the pharmacist, and it is usual to store such medicines out of sight of potential customers so that each request can be noticed and refused if necessary. Where a particular product is known to be subject to misuse, the Royal Pharmaceutical Society's Council has issued a statement to recommend that pharmacists keep written records of sales, including the name and address of purchasers. Examples of products involved include 'Phensedyl' linctus and, more recently, 'Valoid' tablets and 'Marzine' tablets ('Marzine' has since been reformulated to contain cinnarizine rather than cyclizine). 'Migraclear' contains aspirin with cyclizine and its sale should also be carried out personally by the pharmacist.

Ingredients which are known to have been purchased and consumed by addicts include codeine, opiates (usually in the form of tincture of chloroform and morphine or of morphine salts), and sympathomimetic agents such as phenylpropanolomine (which have been used for their stimulant effects as 'substitute amphetamines'). A more extensive list can be found in the current edition of the Royal Pharmaceutical Society's *Medicines and ethics—a guide for the pharmacist.*

Requests for chemicals intended for use in manufacturing or 'cutting' (extending and diluting) illicit drugs might arise in pharmacies. The pharmacist should watch for patterns and clusters of requests for ascorbic acid, citric acid, and glucose (used in 'cutting' heroin), sodium bicarbonate (used in 'crack'), hydrogen peroxide (used in the drug 'ecstasy'), benzyl methyl ketone (a precursor of amphetamine), and amyl nitrite ('poppers').

Pharmacists must be vigilant in controlling sales of solvents liable to abuse and to abide by the Royal Pharmaceutical Society's Council statement on the sale of tobacco which makes the sale of tobacco contrary to the Code of Ethics—that is, unprofessional conduct. Some pharmacies still have a licence for sales of alcohol but it is likely that the Royal Pharmaceutical Society's Council will take steps to address the issue. Pharmacists are already aware that alcohol is the cause of more deaths and domestic misery than any other drug.

12.2 Intravenous drug misuse and the spread of AIDS

World-wide attempts have been made to restrict injecting drug misuse as one means to reduce the spread of the Human Immunodeficiency Virus (HIV). The strategies have included greater attempts to reduce the amount of heroin coming on to the market by paying farmers to grow other crops, by prosecuting the drug traffickers and by attempting to tighten restrictions on entry of drugs through intensifying Customs activities.

The growing concern has been to limit intravenous drug misuse, not only because of its ultimate effects on society but, additionally and more urgently, because of the incontrovertible evidence that intravenous drug misusers are among the major risk groups for HIV infection and AIDS.

Thus, as we have said earlier, strategies have been developed to limit the harm caused by intravenous drug misuse by increasing the supply of clean needles and syringes and also by disseminating information about health. To put the problem in perspective, a major way in which HIV is spread in the heterosexual population in developed countries is by the sharing of injecting equipment among drug users. During 1989 the numbers of heterosexual AIDS cases in the UK increased from 76 to 135, and of heterosexual HIV cases from 517 to 766, while the rate of increase in new cases of HIV infection among homosexual and bisexual men is falling. World-wide, HIV is spread heterosexually by sexual intercourse.

12.3 Supply of injecting equipment from pharmacies

It has always been part of the drug culture that misusers share injecting equipment (their 'works'). For first-time injectors, it will be necessary to borrow somebody else's 'works' to give the first injection. Until recently it has been difficult for drug misusers to buy needles and syringes, and indeed the policy of the Royal Pharmaceutical Society Council, until recent years, was that pharmacists should not sell injecting equipment to drug misusers. It is comparatively recently that this policy was reversed, in recognition of the growing threat from HIV and AIDS.

Traditionally, the sale of injecting equipment has been seen as condoning illegal drug use. We should, therefore, not be surprised that many pharmacists who have been qualified for some time have found the huge shift in attitude and policy difficult to accept. For health professionals, the dilemma between not wishing to encourage illegal drug use while at the same time wanting to prevent the spread of HIV infection has similarly proved to be difficult. For pharmacists who feel there is a moral conflict in this area, we refer them to the opening section of this chapter. In order to limit the global consequences of drug misuse, a United Nations convention requires that all signatory members, such as the United Kingdom, should control certain drugs to make their possession, except in certain limited circumstances, illegal.

In the wake of pilot schemes in Liverpool and Bradford, the concept of needle/syringe exchange schemes through pharmacies became more widely accepted. The Royal Pharmaceutical Society has provided guidelines for pharmacists intending to participate in such schemes (see pp. 192–3). Such schemes are usually organized by the District Health Authority or NHS Regional Health Authority, and funding has now been made available to NHS Regions for projects which are designed to reduce the spread of AIDS, including needle/syringe exchanges. The essential elements of such a scheme are the provision of:

- clean needles and syringes;
- condoms;
- literature about the spread of HIV and AIDS;

- contact numbers for local drug misuse counselling services;
- a safe means of disposal of used equipment.

Participating pharmacies are usually identified by a window sticker and logo, and the local drug agencies are informed of the pharmacies taking part so that they can pass this information to their clients. Recent calls for a nationally-agreed logo have not yet been accepted. Pharmacists are supplied with packs containing clean needles and syringes, and usually condoms and health education material, and also a supply of sharps containers to hand to the drug misuser, who will then place used materials in this container for return to the pharmacy.

All pharmacy staff should be informed that the pharmacy is taking part in the scheme, but only the pharmacist should be involved in dealing with requests for clean equipment and return of used 'works'. However, if the scheme is to be successful, it is important that the staff are clearly informed of the details of the scheme and that requests should be dealt with in a non-judgemental and discreet manner. We would strongly advise the pharmacist to be vaccinated against hepatitis B. The individual sharps containers returned by drug misusers should be placed into an outer container by the drug misuser which would be collected at the request of the pharmacist as part of the scheme. Such collections are generally organized by the Family Health Services Authority, Environmental Health Department or District Health Authority.

12.3.1 Bleach and teach

Drug workers recognize that needle/syringe exchange schemes are a policy of ideals and that, for many reasons, drug misusers will not always return used 'works' or utilize any scheme at all. Recognizing that some drug misusers are likely to continue to re-use, and perhaps to share, their 'works', a second strategy is to have a 'Bleach and Teach' policy. While undoubtedly second-best, this at least can put across the principles of sterilization and cleaning of needles and syringes.

Cleaning injecting equipment will not protect absolutely against HIV infection. The Public Health Laboratory Service advises either:

1. Putting a generous squirt of washing-up liquid into a cup and adding cold water. The liquid should then be drawn up, filling the syringe and then flushed away (not back into the cup). This process should be repeated a second time, then the 'works' flushed through with cold water two or three times.

or

2. Drawing undiluted household bleach to fill the syringe, then flushing it away (not into the container). This procedure should be repeated then the works flushed through with cold water two or three times.

or

3. (The most effective method) Flushing the works through with cold water then immersing needle and syringe in boiling water and boiling for about five minutes. NB: Some syringes do not withstand boiling. Local community drug teams can advise on those which can. Tests have been run by the Public Health Laboratories on most brands, excluding insulin syringes.

12.3.2 Records

While the organizers of needle/syringe exchange schemes are often keen to monitor progress, and thus encourage pharmacists to keep some form of records of clients who use the service, this is not always practicable.

Some pharmacists have attempted to keep rudimentary records using forenames, initials, nicknames, or identifying features for the drug misusers who obtain regular supplies. However, recognizing that drug misusers may well be reluctant to give any information as to their identity, a simple recording of gender and approximate age will suffice. It is important that pharmacists remember that drug misusers perceive a threat of arrest and prosecution for carrying used syringes with their traces of drugs, and that pharmacists tend to be seen as part of the 'Establishment'.

It is often found that the drug misuser will ask for a new supply of 'works' but not return any used needles and syringes. In this sense the term 'exchange' is a misnomer, and it is widely agreed that such supplies should be made with or without the return of used needles and syringes. The media, and sometimes pharmacists themselves, have expressed concern that the wider availability of needles and syringes will lead to an increase in their being discarded indiscriminately and left in public places and in dustbins. While recognizing this concern, to date there is no evidence that this has occurred or that drug misusers are particularly careless in their disposal of sharps. Before the introduction of sharps containers, needles were often disposed of in empty drinks cans, which were then flattened to provide a relatively safe means of disposal, and where no sharps container is available this can be used as a substitute.

Pharmacists should remember that many drug misusers will be crushing tablets and so injecting a slurry rather than the clear solutions that the pharmacist might expect. Thus, in supplying injecting equipment to drug misusers, a range of both needle and syringe sizes should be available. Many needle/syringe exchange schemes contain standard sizes of both in the packs which are to be given out by pharmacists. However, for pharmacists to prepare to deal with requests to buy needles and syringes, local drug agencies are able to provide information about the sizes of needles and syringes used locally and thus which to keep in stock, since in the drug culture this tends to be a 'neighbourhood fashion'. In some areas where previously the disposable 0.5 ml and 1 ml diabetic syringes were the only ones which drug misusers were able to buy, these have become the standard equipment, but this is not invariably the case.

12.4 Manufacturers' response to drug misuse

A range of drugs may be injected intravenously by the misuser, including amphetamines, cocaine, cyclizine, temazepam, barbiturates, and buprenorphine. Pharmacists will remember that the original formulation of 'Marzine' travel sickness tablets contained cyclizine and that a warning was issued to pharmacists that drug misusers were buying large quantities of this product. The tablets were being crushed, dissolved, and injected. A Royal Pharmaceutical Society Council statement appeared recommending that pharmacists made all sales of the product personally and questioned the purchaser to attempt to determine whether the request was genuine. The manufacturer subsequently changed the formulation of the product to include cinnarizine as the active agent, which is not subject to misuse, and apparently this information took some time to filter through to misusers, who continued to purchase it. 'Valoid' tablets still contain cyclizine and their sale must be tightly controlled by the pharmacist. Buprenorphine ('Temgesic') was recently included under Schedule 3 of the Misuse of Drugs legislation, following evidence of misuse, and its prescribing is more tightly controlled. Temazepam capsules originally contained a viscous liquid which was drawn out through the capsule and subsequently injected. However, the manufacturers have responded to concern about the misuse of this drug and the product is now generally available as tablets or as capsules filled with a gel which makes injection difficult.

Drug misusers will move on to new products and substances once restrictions are placed on previous ones, and the pharmacist should be aware of increasing demands for particular over-the-counter products. It will be useful for the pharmacist to maintain contact with local drug agencies, who are likely to know through their outreach workers those drugs and products which are currently being misused.

12.5 Advice from the pharmacist

There are many ways in which pharmacists can promote health by giving advice and information in the area of drug misuse. Firstly, they can continue to participate in the 'Healthcare in the High Street' scheme, stocking and displaying leaflets on relevant topics such as needle/syringe exchange, AIDS, and solvent misuse.

Secondly, they can be a source of information in answer to queries from parents who suspect that their child might be misusing drugs, and from drug misusers themselves.

Thirdly, they can work closely with local agencies working in the field of drug misuse, referring clients for further information and counselling, publicizing the availability of such services, and participating in local campaigns and initiatives. The local Health Promotion Unit can be a valuable source of information and contact points.

12.6 Royal Pharmaceutical Society guidelines for pharmacists involved in schemes to supply clean syringes and needles to addicts

(Published in the *Pharmaceutical Journal*, 11 April 1987) The following guidelines have been approved by the Pharmaceutical Society's Council for the assistance of pharmacists who are, or wish to become, involved in schemes to supply clean syringes and needles to addicts. It should be noted that participation in such schemes is entirely voluntary and at the discretion of the pharmacist involved.

1. The existing facilities should be researched and the pharmacist should liaise with the local pharmaceutical committee (area pharmaceutical committee), local medical committee (area medical committee) and any local drug abuse teams and clinics.

2. It should be established how many pharmacists need to take part, based on how many local drug abusers are actually injecting.

3. The supply of free syringes and needles should always be made by the pharmacist and supplies should always be accompanied by advice and encouragement to make use of any local drug advisory services. Any leaflets from health education agencies, local drug dependency clinics, or 'walk-in centres' should be available.

4. All persons requesting free syringes and needles should be encouraged to surrender used equipment to a designated centre.

5. Disposal of dirty syringes and needles should be through a recognized sharps disposal system. Some health authorities or family practitioner committees (health boards) may be prepared to channel collections into the service offered to general practitioners or offer additional resources to operate the exchange scheme. Rentokil offers a suitable alternative.

6. Returned syringes and needles should be put straight into the sharps disposal box by the user. In a pharmacy this box should be stored in a secure place and made available to the user who wishes to deposit syringes and needles. Addicts should be en-

couraged to place dirty syringes and needles in an outer container before placing them in the sharps disposal box. It should not be necessary for any member of staff to handle any dirty syringes or needles.

Contact points

The Royal Pharmaceutical Society's Inspector and the local Drug Squad officer, both of whom make regular visits and inspect the Controlled Drugs registers, are familiar with the local drug 'scene' and are valuable sources of information and advice.

Standing Conference on Drug Abuse (SCODA) is the national coordinating body for voluntary organisations/ agencies working in the field of drug misuse. Pharmacists can contact them to obtain details of local groups.

Appendix 1 Key points

Stopping smoking

Key counselling times

- When customers ask about anti-smoking products
- When smokers present with coughs
- When a smoker is pregnant

Key advice points

- Choose a day to stop (one when there is likely to be as little stress as possible)
- Tell everyone you are going to stop, enlist moral support
- Get rid of the paraphernalia of smoking—ashtrays, lighters, cigarettes
- On the chosen day, stop smoking
- Work on staying stopped, come back to the pharmacy each week to discuss progress

'Nicorette'—key points

- 'Nicorette' should not be chewed like ordinary gum
- It will not work if the content is swallowed
- The stick of gum should be chewed six to ten times then 'parked' against the gum, between gum and cheek
- This will allow the nicotine to be absorbed through the buccal mucosa
- Side-effects may include minor stomach upset, sore mouth, and belching

Alcohol

Units of alcohol

1 Unit = 1 glass wine
½ pint bitter, cider, standard lager
1 pub measure of spirits (gin, whisky, etc.)
1 pub measure sherry or vermouth

Points to remember

- 'Extra strength' lagers have a higher alcohol content

- Home-poured measures of spirits are generally larger than the standard pub measure

- 'Low-alcohol' beers and wines are not 'no-alcohol'—check the alcohol content by per cent volume

- There is no 'safe driving' limit. Reaction times and blood alcohol levels vary between individuals even when the same amount of alcohol is drunk

- Maximum drinking limits for good health are
14 units per week for women
21 units per week for men

- Medicines and alcohol—caution with hypnotics, tranquillizers, antihistamines, anticonvulsants, moderate to strong analgesics, metronidazole (disulfiram-type reaction)

Healthy eating

Key changes for everyone

- Eat less fat, especially saturated fat
- Eat more fibre, especially by eating more fruit and vegetables
- Eat less sugar
- Eat less salt
- Drink less alcohol

Lowering cholesterol

The amount of cholesterol in the blood is not simply determined by eating foods which contain cholesterol. Eating saturated fats (animal fats) influences the amount of cholesterol in the blood. Eating a diet which is low in fat and particularly low in saturated fat can help to reduce cholesterol levels.

Eating a low-fat diet generally leads to weight loss. Not everyone who wants to lower their blood cholesterol will want to lose weight. Maintaining calorie intake but with less saturated fat will be their goal. Others will need to lose weight and guidelines are given below.

Ways to reduce fat in the diet

- Change from full-fat to semi-skimmed or skimmed milk
- Eat less red meat and choose lean cuts
- Eat more chicken, turkey, and fish
- Grill rather than fry foods
- If frying, use vegetable oils rather than animal fats such as lard
- Change from butter or standard margarine to a spread containing polyunsaturates
- Low-fat versions of polyunsaturate spreads are available

Dietary changes for losing weight

- Eat a low-fat diet, following the guidelines above
- Change to low-fat milk and low-fat polyunsaturate spread
- Change to low-fat cheeses (cut down the amount of hard cheese eaten, eat more cottage cheese, and watch fat content of others)
- If sweet foods and drinks are still preferred, choose ones with sweet substitutes for sugar
- Eat more fresh fruit and green vegetables
- As well as dietary change, take more exercise (about 20 minutes, two or three times a week)

Baby and child health

Vaccination schedules

2, 3, and 4 months	Diphtheria, tetanus, pertussis (DTP), and polio
12–18 months	Measles, mumps, rubella
4–5 years	Booster diphtheria, tetanus, polio
10–14 years	Rubella (girls only)
10–14 years	BCG (interval of 3 weeks between BCG and rubella)
15–18 years	Booster tetanus and polio

Paracetamol and young babies

Paracetamol can be given to babies under three months old for mild febrile reactions associated with the first dose of DTP vaccine. The standard dose is 5–10 mg/kg.

Infant feeding

Benefits of breast-feeding

- Inexpensive

- Protects baby against gastroenteritis and other infections

- Bonding between mother and baby

- May protect against development of allergies in later life

Cow's milk and babies

- Full-fat cow's milk should not be given to babies under one year old

- Nutritionally, unmodified cow's milk is unsuitable for young babies and may lead to allergies

- Semi-skimmed cow's milk should not be given to children aged under two years

- Skimmed cow's milk should not be given to children aged under five

- The low-fat milks do not contain sufficient fat-soluble vitamins and are low in calories.

Appendix 2 Contact points

Chapter 4

British Heart Foundation (BHF), 102 Gloucester Place, London W1H 4DH. Tel. 071 935 0185. BHF has a wide range of publications and information sources on coronary heart disease and has an active educational role for both health professionals and the public.
Coronary Prevention Group (CPG), 60 Great Ormond Street, London WC1N 3HR. Tel. 071 833 3687. CPG has an extensive range of literature and a telephone enquiry service.
Family Heart Association (FHA), PO Box 116, Kidlington, Oxford OX5 1DT. Tel. 0865 779125. FHA aims to increase awareness about familial hyperlipidaemias and has been involved in devising guidelines for cholesterol testing.
Health Education Authority (HEA), Hamilton House, Mableden Place, London WC1H 9TX. Tel. 071 383 3833.

Chapter 5

For advice and guidance on setting-up and maintaining screening and testing services in a pharmacy:
Royal Pharmaceutical Society of Great Britain, 1 Lambeth High Street, London SE1 7JN. Tel. 071 735 9141.
National Pharmaceutical Association, Mallinson House, 40–42 St Peter's Street, St Albans, Herts AL1 3NP. Tel. 0727 832161.
Pharmaceutical Services Negotiating Committee, 59 Buckingham Street, Aylesbury, Bucks HP20 2PJ. Tel. 0296 392181.

Chapter 6

British Association of Cancer United Patients (BACUP), 121–123 Charterhouse Street, London EC1M 6AA. Tel. 071 608 1661. Booklets, fact sheets, information for health professionals, patients, and their relatives. Tel. Freephone 0800 181199 for telephone enquiries and counselling service.

Cancer Link, 17 Britannia Street, London WC1 9JN. Tel. 071 833 2451. Patient support groups, information.
Cancer Research Campaign, 2 Carlton House Terrace, London SW1Y 5AR. Tel. 071 930 8972. Information, leaflets, and other educational materials.
Imperial Cancer Research Fund, PO Box 123, Lincoln's Inn Fields, London WC2A 3PX. Tel. 071 242 0200.

Chapter 7

Action on Smoking and Health (ASH), 5–11 Mortimer Street, London W1N 7RH. Tel. 071 637 9843.
British Medical Acupuncture Society, 67–69 Chancery Lane, London WC2 1AF.
British Society of Medical and Dental Hypnosis, 42 Links Road, Ashtead, Surrey KT21 2HJ.
Health Education Authority (see contact points for Chapter 4).
QUIT (formerly National Association of Non-smokers), Latimer House, 40–48 Hanson Street, London W1P 7DE. Tel. 071 636 9103 or QUITLINE 071 323 0505.

Chapter 8

Alcoholics Anonymous, General Service Office. PO Box 1, Stonebow House, York YO1 2NJ. Tel. 0904 644026/7/8/9.
Aquarius, 6th Floor, The White House, 111 New Street, Birmingham B2 4EU Tel. 021 632 4727.

Chapter 9

British Dietetic Association, Daimler House, Paradise Circus, Queensway, Birmingham B1 2BJ. Tel. 021 643 5483.
Health Education Authority (see contact points for Chapter 4).

Chapter 10

Enuresis Research and Information Council, 65 St Michael's Hill, Bristol BS2 8ZD. Tel. 0272 264920. For further information, send a stamped addressed envelope.

Chapter 11

Family Planning Information Service, 27–35 Mortimer Street, London W1N 7RJ. Tel. 071 636 7866. Provides a nationwide telephone enquiry service, leaflets on all methods of contraception, and other useful information in the field of sexual and reproductive health. Also runs the Healthwise bookshop (see p. 205).

Chapter 12

The Royal Pharmaceutical Society's Inspector and the local Drug Squad officer, both of whom make regular visits and inspect the Controlled Drugs registers, are familiar with the local drug scene and are valuable sources of information and advice.

Standing Conference on Drug Abuse (SCODA), 1–4 Hatton Place, London EC1 8ND. Tel. 071 430 2341. SCODA is the national coordinating body for voluntary organizations and agencies working in the field of drug misuse. Pharmacists can contact them to obtain details of local groups.

Institute for the Study of Drug Dependence (ISDD) same address as SCODA. They can provide useful information and also publish a bimonthly magazine on drug dependence, Druglink, for those working in the field.

Further reading

Chapter 1

Acheson, R. M. and Hagard, S. (1984). *Health, society and medicine—an introduction to community medicine*. Blackwell Scientific Publications, Oxford.

Ewles, L. and Simnett, I. (1985). *Promoting health—a practical guide to health education*. John Wiley & Sons, Chichester.

Muir-Gray, J. (1979). *Man against disease*. Oxford University Press, Oxford.

Townsend, P., Davidson, N., and Whitehead, M. (1988). *Inequalities in health (the* Black report *and* The health divide). Penguin, London.

Smith, A. and Jacobson, B. (ed.) (1988). *The nation's health—a strategy for the 1990s*. Health Education Authority, London School of Hygiene and Tropical Medicine, and King Edward's Hospital Fund for London, London.

Smith, R. (1987). *Unemployment and health—a disaster and a challenge*. Oxford University Press, Oxford.

Chapter 2

Harris, J. (1986). *Smoking and the community pharmacist*. Academic Department of Community medicine, King's College Hospital Medical School, London.

HMSO (1987). *Promoting better health*. HMSO, London.

Nuffield Foundation (1986). *Pharmacy: the report of a Committee of Inquiry*. The Nuffield Foundation, London.

Panton, R. S. and Blenkinsopp, A. (1989). *Stop smoking—pharmacy action*. West Midlands Regional Health Authority, (Regional Pharmacy Office), Birmingham.

Pauncefort, Z. and Zeelenburg, S. (1989). *Pharmacy healthcare*. Family Planning Association, London.

Shafford, A. and Sharpe, K. (1989). *The pharmacist as a health educator*. Health Education Authority, London.

Chapter 3

Burnard, P. (1989). *Counselling skills for health professionals.* Chapman & Hall, London.
Ewles, L. and Simnett, I. (*see* further reading for Chapter 1).
Hargie, O. (ed.) (1986). *A handbook of communication skills.* Croom Helm, Beckenham, Kent.
Hargie, O., Saunders, C., and Dickson, D. (1987). *Social skills in interpersonal communication.* Croom Helm, Beckenham, Kent.
Kitching, J. B. and Jones, I. F. (1990). Communicating with patients. Pharmaceutical Journal series published during 1990.
Ley, P. (1988). *Communicating with patients.* Croom Helm, Beckenham, Kent.
Morrow, N. C. and Hargie, O., Interpersonal communication. *Pharmacy Update* article series published during 1985 and 1987.
Tindall, W., Beardsley, R. S., and Kimberlin, C. L. (1989). *Communication skills in pharmacy practice.* Lea and Febiger.

Chapter 4

Acheson, R. M. and Hagard, S. (*see* further reading for Chapter 1).
Fowler, G. (1983). *Practising prevention.* British Medical Association, London.
HEA (1987). *Broken hearts: the cost of coronary heart disease in England.* Health Education Authority, London.
National Forum for Coronary Heart Disease Prevention (1988). *Coronary heart disease prevention—action in the UK 1984–1987.* Health Education Authority, London.
Smith, A. and Jacobson, B. (*see* further reading for Chapter 1).

Chapter 5

Royal Pharmaceutical Society, Law Department (1990). *Medicines, ethics and practice—a guide for pharmacists.* Pharmaceutical Press, London.
Fowler, G. (*see* further reading for Chapter 4).

Chapter 6

Austoker, J. and Humphreys, J. (1988). *Breast cancer screening.* Oxford University Press, Oxford.
Doll, R. and Peto, R. (1981). *The causes of cancer.* Oxford University Press, Oxford.
Heller, T., Davey, B. and Bailey, L. (ed.) (1989). *Reducing the risk of cancers.* The Open University, Hodder and Stoughton, London.

Chapter 7

Ashton, H. and Stepney, R. (1982). *Smoking: psychology and pharmacology*. Tavistock Publications, London.
Royal College of Physicians (1978). *Smoking and health*. Pitman Medical, London.
Royal College of Physicians (1983). *Health or smoking*. Pitman Medical, London.
Taylor, P. (1984). *Smoking: the politics of tobacco*. Bodley Head, London.
WHO/BMA. *Smoke-free Europe—1. The physicians role. 3. The evaluation and monitoring of public action on tobacco. 4. Tobacco or health. 7. The dying of the light* and *9. Tobacco price and the smoking epidemic.*

Chapter 8

Royal College of Physicians (1987). *The medical consequences of alcohol abuse*. Tavistock Publications, London.
Royal College of Psychiatrists (1986). *Alcohol—our favourite drug*. Tavistock Publications, London.

Chapter 9

Committee on Medical Aspects of Food Policy (1984). *Diet and Cardiovascular disease*. HMSO, London.
Committee on Medical Aspects of Food Policy (1989). *Dietary sugars and human disease*. HMSO, London.
Consumers' Association (1989). *Healthy eating—fact and fiction*. Hodder and Stoughton, London.
National Advisory Committee on Nutritional Education (1983). *Proposals for nutritional guidelines for health education in Britain*. Health Education Council, London.
Royal College of Physicians (1980). *Medical aspects of dietary fibre*. Pitman Medical, London.
WHO (1988). *Nutrition and health.*
Yetiv, J. (1986). *Sense and nonsense in nutrition*. Penguin, London.

Chapter 10

Committee on Medical Aspects of Food Policy (1988). *Present-day practice in infant feeding* (third report). HMSO, London.
HMSO (1990). *Immunisation against infectious diseases.*
Modell, M. and Boyd, R. (1988). *Paediatric problems in general practice* (2nd edn). Oxford University Press, Oxford.

Valman, H. B. (1989). *The first year of life*, (3rd edn). British Medical Association, London.
Valman, H. B. (1988). *ABC of one to seven*, (2nd edn). British Medical Association, London.

Chapter 11

Flynn, A. and Brooks, M. (1988). *Manual of natural family planning*. Unwin-Hyman, London.
Guillebaud, J. (1989). *Contraception—your questions answered*. Pitman Medical, London.
Guillebaud, J. (1989). *The pill*. Oxford University Press, Oxford.
Kilmartin, A. (1989). *Understanding cystitis*. Arrow Books.
McPherson, A. (ed.) (1988). *Women's problems in general practice*. Oxford University Press, Oxford.
Healthwise, the Family Planning Association's bookshop stocks all the above books and others in this field (27–35 Mortimer Street, London W1N 7RJ. Tel. 071 636 7866).

Chapter 12

Banks, A. and Waller, T. A. N. (1988). *Drug misuse—a practical handbook for GPs*. Blackwell Scientific Publications, Oxford.
Continuing Education Centre (1988). *AIDS now—some questions answered*. Leicester Polytechnic.
Dale, J. R. and Appelbe, G. (1989). *Pharmacy law and ethics*. Pharmaceutical Press, London.
Glanz, A., Byrne, C., and Jackson, P. (1990). *Prevention of AIDS among drug misusers: the role of the high street pharmacy*. Institute of Psychiatry, London.
Maddock, H. (1987). *Drug abuse*. Pharmaceutical Press, London.
Medicines and ethics—a guide for pharmacists (1990). Pharmaceutical Press, London.
Tyler, A. (1989). *Street drugs*. New English Library.
WHO (1986). *Drug dependence and alcohol-related problems: a manual for community health workers*.

Index